WHAT PEOPLE ARE SAYING ABOUT

BECOME YOUR OWN DOCTOR

Classical and Renaissance physicians regarded food as medicine. Paul Lloyd revives their ancient science in his guidebook for healthy eating based on understanding the four humoral types: choleric, sanguine, melancholic and phlegmatic. Different foods can have positive or negative effects, and Lloyd explains how to find the right balance for optimal health. He includes tried-and-tested recipes utilizing common household and garden ingredients to treat a range of ailments according to humoral principles. Paul Lloyd has tapped into a cornucopia of wisdom that we can apply in these modern times of conflicting health advice.

Ruth Parnell, subeditor and book reviewer, *NEXUS Magazine*

Become Your Own Doctor

Lost Secrets of Humoral Healthcare Revealed

Become Your Own Doctor

Lost Secrets of Humoral Healthcare Revealed

Paul Lloyd

AYNI BOOKS

Winchester, UK
Washington, USA

First published by Ayni Books, 2016
Ayni Books is an imprint of John Hunt Publishing Ltd., Laurel House, Station Approach,
Alresford, Hants, SO24 9JH, UK
office1@jhpbooks.net
www.johnhuntpublishing.com
www.ayni-books.com

For distributor details and how to order please visit the 'Ordering' section on our website.

ISBN: 978 1 78535 390 1
Library of Congress Control Number: 2016931746

A CIP catalogue record for this book is available from the British Library.

Design: Stuart Davies

Printed and bound by CPI Group (UK) Ltd, Croydon, CR0 4YY, UK

We operate a distinctive and ethical publishing philosophy in all
areas of our business, from our global network of authors to
production and worldwide distribution.

CONTENTS

To the memory of Barbara Hazel Wellstood and
Francis Kenneth Lloyd

Introduction

In the latter part of 2014, between finishing my book *Food and Identity in England* and starting my next university teaching assignment, I wrote a two-part article on alternative medicine for *Nexus Magazine*. In discussing the history of an ancient and time-honored medical theory and practice known as humorism, I showed briefly how this might be applied to modern-day living. Following the article's publication in April and June 2015 I received many messages from interested readers who wanted to know more about humorism and medical self-help. Clearly there was enough interest for me to expand on the topic, both in breadth and depth, by writing this book for the benefit of a wide audience.

But what was new to say on the topic? After all, in recent years many works have been published on "alternative medicine" – a term that is sometimes used in a derogatory way by some doctors, but thankfully not all of them, who either ignore or choose to forget the roots of their own practice. These works on how to cure illnesses and how to prevent them from occurring in the first place, which, thanks to the internet, have been inspired by increased public awareness of medical matters and a growing interest in taking control personally over one's own healthcare, include instructing readers on how to make and administer herbal remedies. While these books are immensely valuable, they convey only part of the story of healthcare at home. This book is different. In recognizing the stark reality that highly trained medical experts in ancient times recognized – that *all* foods, not just herbs, have essential medicinal properties, and that our choice in foods is *the* major factor in preventing and curing illnesses – I unlock the treasure chest of bygone humoral wisdom and discuss home-made medicine and personal healthcare in a broad way.

Let me make it clear from the outset that this book does not intend to critique the modern medical profession. Few people would be rash enough to doubt the very real progress that has been facilitated by scientific research in recent years. Similarly, it seems obvious that modern nutritional theory is helping some people to live longer. To people outside the medical profession, however, it is equally obvious that the latest advice (whatever that currently may be) is not, and never has been, the final word of wisdom. Conflicting advice is everywhere we look with one group of researchers questioning the findings of another. Foods that were considered conducive to good health not long ago must, we are told, be deleted from our diets right now if we are to avoid diabetes / cancer / heart attacks, etc. As we all know, sugar – considered to be a pillar of healthfulness in the early to mid-twentieth century – is one such food that has lost favor with dieticians. Alcoholic beverages taken in small quantities are good for one's health, or bad for it, depending on which researchers you choose to believe; fresh fruit, a one-time inducer of all manner of ills, is considered essential – at least for now; and "processed meats do cause cancer" according to a recent World Health Organization report that also says meat has "health benefits," and, in the next breath, trumpets the notion that eating "two slices of bacon" could be dangerous (http://www.bbc.co.uk/news/health-34615621). We are told to eat plenty of fiber; sound advice, one might suppose, but how long will it be before this pearl of wisdom is consigned by researchers to the dustbin of medical history because some future study or another declares that fiber can cause health problems? There clearly has never been a better time to reappraise where we are going by looking back at where we have come from. In so doing, we might feel that there is much to gain by adopting a back-to-basics approach to daily regimen and medicine, and at once circumvent the need to wait an increasingly inordinate length of time to consult our hard-pressed general practitioners.

Prior to physicians, apothecaries and drug manufacturers adopting mineral and chemical compounds to cure health problems, which, cynics claim, were introduced to mystify the medical profession and justify practitioners' wealth and prestige, effective healthcare was based on an ancient system known as *humorism*. Within this system the body was at one with its natural environment, and bodily imbalances that brought on disease were rectified by the patient (or his or her carer) applying a set of complex but easily understandable rules. We are told by many of today's doctors that medicine has moved on since then, and that we should trust the latest (and often controversial and/or contradictory) advice pushed by scientists and their young research assistants keen to convince us that they are the new holders of the ultimate truth. They claim we are fitter than ever before, and in any case, they say, there is no scientific evidence that half of the humors actually exist. But does this ancient medical knowledge lose its validity because of its age – even though wise sages who practiced it in antiquity had a complex (and accurate) knowledge of mathematics and astronomy, and bequeathed to us also the calendar, time measurement, bookkeeping, law-making and civic society? Is humorism unsound because some humors can neither be found nor measured by scientists? If this is so, why should we be asked to believe in astrophysicists' "dark matter" and cosmologists' "singularity" – neither of which have been proven to exist? Whether or not the humors "kholé" and "melas kholé" can actually be located and identified, the bottom line is that humorism was finely tuned and its medicines were used – and used successfully according to a vast number of letters, diaries and notebooks – to treat all kinds of ailments for centuries. These handwritten testaments are available for everyone to see at city and county record offices; I know because I have studied hundreds of them.

Modern medical/dietary advice seems to suggest that, like a

pair of stretchy socks or spandex shorts with an elasticated waistband, one size fits all: We should cut down on sugar consumption, researchers tell us. Undoubtedly this is true in some cases; but this sweeping statement apparently ignores an individual's medical condition. Another abstraction resulting from a medical study relates to the healthfulness of eating copious amounts of fruit and vegetables (which ironically contain sugar, but the good news, we are told, is that it is the right sort of sugar!). These foods are so advantageous, they say, we should all eat at least "five a day." On the basis of current wisdom this may be sound advice to many, but tell that to people who have had a carcinoid and part of their intestines removed! The generalizations go on… In our headlong rush to embrace new ideas and to accept every scrap of subjective medical/dietary advice as gospel, we have lost touch with traditional humoral-based healthcare that, assuredly and correctly, recognizes that one size certainly does not fit all. This book, like those published by doctors before the advent of chemical medicines, recognizes that our bodily requirements are individual, and that they can be maintained with the aid of individualistically tailored diets and easily made medicines. Indeed, reading a newspaper this morning, it seems that a few enlightened scientific researchers might agree with me as modern research, at long last, starts to catch up with ancient humoral knowledge regarding the health benefits of personalized diets (see: http://well.blogs.nytimes.com/2016/01/11/a-personalized-diet-better-suited-to-you/?smid=fb-share&_r=0).

In the first chapter I offer the reader a brief history of humorism, describing the nature of the humoral body and medicine, and discussing why for centuries it was so important in maintaining good health and preventing illnesses. I will look at its revival in Renaissance Europe and reveal some of the reasons for its enduring resilience in the face of challenges from those who thought the answer to humanity's health problems lay in taking chemical and mineral compounds orally and applying them externally to everything from wounds to blemishes. Traditionalists who had good reason to believe that their health had been maintained effectively by eating the right foods and supplementing this by taking organic medicines, however, needed to understand their own peculiar bodily requirements in humoral terms. This was not incomprehensible science to our ancestors, and for us to embrace the theory and practice of health through humorism we must first recognize our own complexions and needs. This aspect of managing one's own healthcare is addressed in Chapter Two, "Recognizing Your Own Bodily Imbalance." I show my readers the signs to look for so that they can determine their own broad humoral makeup, and I explain how one can fine-tune this knowledge and use it to decide on the best lifestyle choices, dietary regimes and appropriate medicines in order to gain from improving one's health.

Whatever a person's humoral complexion might be, finding the right foods to maintain good health or to combat illness is not a problem. Whether one is a vegetarian or a red-blooded meat eater, or whether one has a preference for fish, fruit, cheese or eggs, optimal wellbeing is a question of performing a balancing act; thus Chapters Three to Seven discuss the attributes of a range of foods in turn. It will be seen that while several foods can be used to fight a specific illness, some might be more suitable than others depending on the patient's humoral temperament and physical and mental disposition. Chapters Three and Four consider the properties and values of a broad range of common fresh fruits, herbs and vegetables. In addition to making nutritious and tasty primary ingredients in meals suitable for vegetarians and non-vegetarians alike, these foods have a wide variety of humoral qualities that enable the diner to achieve the ideal balance for his or her own particular need. It will be seen that these foods are also the most likely ones to be turned into medicines to treat a broad range of maladies. Another genre of foodstuffs that is ideal as ingredients in meals – not only from the point of view of subtly enhancing taste, texture and color, but also from the aspect of rectifying humoral imbalance – is the one that incorporates spices, condiments and dried fruits. These ingredients are discussed in Chapter Five. Usually but not always taking a supplementary role in meals, they differ from many foods in the herbs and fresh fruit category in that, as will be explained, they are often humorally "warmer" and "dryer" than the latter. Consequently they are extremely valuable for treating a different range of medical conditions.

In the sixth and seventh chapters I turn my attention to the specific humoral qualities and medical attributes of a range of foods commonly found in butchers' shops, dairy stores, and on fishmongers' and poulterers' market stalls. The reasons for wanting or needing to abstain from eating flesh or other products sourced from animals are many and varied, and include, of course, an admirable concern for the welfare of our fellow creatures. These people are known as "vegans" or "vegetarians," but some of them – perhaps more accurately describable as "vegaquarians" – eat fish. Whether or not one chooses to eat fish, meat or poultry, or whether one lives on fruits and vegetables, one can achieve nutritional balance and optimal health by adjusting one's intake to suit one's own personal requirements at any given time. Different sorts of flesh have humoral character-istics that should not be overlooked, however. As is the case for the other foodstuffs mentioned above, whether one is male or female, young or old, active of sedentary, fit or ill, there is a broad range of meats available to service every humoral complexion, to provide variety, and to suit all medical/dietary requirements.

The eighth and final chapter looks at advice handed down to us on how to make a range of medicines that can be used both to protect the members of the household from contracting illnesses and to help cure existing ones. This chapter discusses also the perceived values of home-made lotions which may be applied to the skin to treat wounds, blemishes and bites. It will be seen that making lotions and potions does not need to be complicated for them to be effective, and that this aspect of healthcare at home is just one part of an overall procedure that can be tailored to suit individual requirements. Let us start by looking at the maintenance and restoration of bodily and mental health at a time when "alternative" medicine was mainstream.

Part I – Humorism

Chapter One

When "Alternative" Medicine
was Mainstream

There was a time when the practice now known as "alternative" medicine was, in fact, mainstream. Everyone from highly qualified doctors to amateur healers, and from clerics and high-ranking lords to lowly peasants, understood the needs of the body in terms of its relationship with the environment; and people who kept diaries and notebooks were convinced that humoral-based medicines worked very well indeed. In order to comprehend the workings of this system we need to start by briefly looking at the history of humorism. In this chapter I look at its roots and revival in Renaissance Europe and reveal some of the reasons for its enduring resilience in the face of challenges from those who thought the answer to humanity's health problems lay in taking chemicals and minerals orally, and in applying them externally to treat skin complaints. I describe the nature of humorism, the humoral body and medicine, and reveal why, for centuries, humoral treatments were so important in maintaining good health and preventing illnesses.

Before more "scientific" ideas were adopted by doctors, starting with the chemical and mechanical body theories forwarded by pioneers such as Swiss alchemist Paracelsus – which supposedly necessitate the use of chemicals, minerals and distillates to cure illnesses *introduced* to the body – our ancestors up until around the mid-1600s clearly understood wellbeing in quite another way. Prevention and cure of illnesses that originated *within* the body, learned people knew, was part of the same package that had at its core respecting the so-called "non-naturals." These are breathing in high-quality, non-polluted air; regular and timely evacuation of bladder and bowel; correct and adequate exercise; sleeping soundly; avoiding perturbation of the mind such as stressful thoughts and bad dreams; and, most importantly – because it was clearly understood that food *is* medicine – eating and drinking the right foods in the right quantities at the right time. Thus, lifestyle is key; and, as physician James Hart who in 1633 wrote a book called *Klinike* observed, this means eating humorally balanced meals. Hart was just one of many doctors who thought along these lines, for this theory had become established among medical experts and accepted by the public who applied this wisdom at the point of treatment. So where did the ideas come from?

They appear to have been known and used by people living in ancient Greece and classical Rome, but they are probably rooted in much earlier civilizations. This can be seen in the works of two ancients: Claudius Galen, a well-respected physician and philosopher who was born in Turkey and lived in Greece, Alexandria and Rome between AD 130 and AD 210; and "the father of Western medicine" Hippocrates who lived in Greece six centuries earlier. Even in Hippocrates' time, which was four hundred years before Jesus was born, there was nothing new in humoral medicine, for this insightful and well-informed Greek physician – who bequeathed to us the still-important Hippocratic Oath – insisted that *his* medical knowledge was ancient even at that time. Thus, it is probable that humorism was received indirectly from exceptionally knowledgeable sages inhabiting Mesopotamia in the earliest of times – wise men who also passed down to us advanced mathematics, accurate astronomy, writing, accountancy, recordkeeping, libraries, law-making and rules for living a harmonious life within the framework of civic society.

During the Renaissance period in Europe (circa 1300 to 1650) there was a revival of interest in all things Greek and Roman, and this included art, architecture, literature and science – including medicine. Thus, the works of Galen and Hippocrates came to occupy a central position in the medical theories of late medieval and early modern physicians. Given that the Roman Empire was centered in the country that is now known as Italy, it is perhaps unsurprising that this country's humanist scholars were at the cutting edge of reviving and analyzing classical teachings. It is equally unsurprising to find the main Renaissance medical training facility here. Prior to Montpellier in Southern France becoming the main European center for medical students, the School of Medicine at Salerno, close to Naples in Southern Italy's Campania region, was *the* distinguished medical teaching facility. So much so that it attracted scholars from all over Europe. Here students learned about the theories of great thinkers who had lived in the dim and distant past – how best to cure illnesses, and even how to help prevent them from occurring in the first place – and, with critical eyes, they adapted them to suit their own environmental conditions and relatively modern ways of life. It was largely the words of wisdom of these Southern European scholars that informed the writings of medical practitioners in Northern Europe, Britain and, subsequently, North America.

So what was the nature of this medical knowledge that was readopted by physicians in the Middle Ages? Doctors based their advice on the firm belief that good health depends on achieving a fine balance between the four humors present in the body. These are black bile, yellow bile, phlegm, and "particles" located within blood. Any imbalance, no matter how small, results in the body becoming too dry or damp, or too cool or warm. This imbalance, they showed through observation and experimentation, can then cause mental or physical health problems. The rationale of doctors' convictions was clear: because all organic matter contains the same humors, but in different forms and amounts, it logically follows that each type of food has its own specific humoral properties. These humors are transferred to the body when the food is eaten, so a diet that improves one's health can be selected. There is no need for chemically produced medicine, experts understood, because food *is* medicine. Illnesses accordingly require short-term dietary adjustment; and books called "dietaries," written by doctors and pharmacists, served as useful guides to healthful living.

Accomplished, qualified medical professionals understood clearly that choosing the right diet was central to maintaining good health; but they also knew that the other "non-naturals" (lifestyle choices) helped. Then as now, sufficient rest, good-quality sleep, sufficient exercise and stress management were considered important under the humoral philosophy; thus books known as "regimen manuals" were also published. These were more comprehensive. Some dietaries and regimen guidebooks were written for the benefit of medical scholars. These contained in-depth advice in technical language; examples include Gualtherus Bruele's *Praxis medicinae* (1628) and Dr Thomas Moffett's *Healths Improvement* (1655). Shorter books written in simple terms were aimed at unqualified people who had an interest in healthcare. An example of these is Philip Moore's *The Hope of Health* (1564). Both dietaries and regimen guidebooks usually contain gender- and age-specific advice; and, because specific foods are key to adjusting health, *all* of them include sections on foods' humoral properties.

What are these properties? Each person and each type of food was known by medical experts to be comprised of the two basic humoral qualities – namely heat and moisture. One can be either temperate (neutral), hot and dry, cold and dry, hot and moist, or cold and moist. Furthermore, heat and moisture each have nine stations (known as "degrees"); these range from hot in the fourth degree (very hot) through temperate to cold in the fourth degree (very cold), and the same for moisture (very dry to very moist). Thus a person or type of food can occupy any one of 81 stations (9 x 9). In addition to the "temperate" stations where there is no excess in heat or cold, or no superfluous dryness or moisture, there are 16 shades of hot and dry (4 x 4), and 16 each of cold and dry, hot and moist, and cold and moist. In practical terms – expressed somewhat simplistically – food additives with opposing humoral properties to the main ingredient can help to neutralize a dish, and a meal with opposing humoral properties to its consumer can be eaten to help rectify his or her humoral imbalance.

It is important to realize that when doctors discuss humoral "heat" and "moisture," they are not referring to physical temperature, or to dryness or dampness in the sense that you can feel it. If this was the case a freshly cooked joint of beef taken straight out of the oven would be humorally "warmer" than a refrigerated joint of lamb. It is not. Similarly, one might expect hard cheese to be humorally "dryer" than cream cheese. Again, this is not the case. As doctors explain, it is all about humors – and these are discussed at length below.

In addition to informing their readers about the benefits of certain foods, and about the harm they can do, some dietaries even subdivide each degree into three further parts. With the seasons of the year and climatic conditions also affecting a person's humors, this level of detail helps to fine-tune the body as and when required.

So what do ancient and Renaissance medical experts mean when they write about "humors"? And how are humors understood to affect health? Sir Thomas Elyot, a renowned sixteenth-century scholar who had a thirst for knowledge and a keen interest in medicine, describes them in this way: The blood humor holds a pre-eminent position over the other three. Because it is moderate in heat and moisture, it preserves the body. Distemperature of blood occurs when one, or more, of the other three humors either becomes excessive or mixes with (and pollutes) the others. Another humor is in phlegm. There are, he said, two sorts of phlegm – natural and unnatural. Natural phlegm is cold and moist, white and tasteless. Containing mainly water, it is produced when digestion is slow and partial. Thus, the goodness cannot be converted to heat-generating blood. Natural phlegm is fine when the right quantity is in the body, but too much of it can result in illness. Unnatural phlegm is that which is mixed with, and has been texturally altered by, other humors. Its characteristics typically are these: colorless, green or chalky; it is thick, slimy and viscose; it is cold; and it is either salt or sour. Again, too much of this unnatural humor is dangerous.

The third humor is known as choler or yellow bile. This is also of two kinds – natural and unnatural. The former sort is clear red or orange in color, and is hot and dry. It is, Elyot says, "engendered of the most subtle part of matter decoct, or boiled in the stomach, whose beginning is in the liver." This is an important bodily element, but an excessive amount dries the constitution, which is particularly detrimental to the wellbeing of physically active people. Unnatural choler is that which is "mixed or corrupted with other humours," and its characteristics are of four sorts: yellow – being a mixture of natural choler and the phlegm humor, with less heat than pure choler; yellowy orange – being a mixture of natural choler and the humor found in congealed phlegm; a light green sort that originates in the stomach rather than in the liver; and a darker green sort that is poisonous. The humor known as black bile, sometimes referred to as black choler or melancholy, also comes in two kinds. The natural sort, Elyot believed, comes from the dregs of pure blood, and can be recognized by its blackness when "it issueth either downward or upward." It is cold and dry; and although in the right quantity it is essential in maintaining good health, too much of it can induce despondency and can leave the body susceptible to contracting disease. The unnatural kind, which is produced in the body as a result of a corruption of choleric yellow bile, is hotter and lighter. This unnatural bile is particularly dangerous to mental health because it can induce low spirits, despondency and feelings of dejection that can result in depression.

The humoral station of male manual workers is understood to be slightly hot and dry, hence their need to drink copious quantities of fluids. If a man or a woman is overly hot and dry, he or she is said to have a "choleric" complexion. This means that there is too much yellow bile, or corrupted choler, in the body. One of the many signs of this is restlessness; another is feistiness. In order to rectify this condition, and to avoid the possibility of leaving the person susceptible to contracting the sorts of illness described below, he or she would be advised to adjust his or her diet to include more humorally cool, moist ingredients – such as certain types of vegetables or fruits – in order to achieve equilibrium.

In comparison to men, it is understood that women in general terms (although not always) are slightly to the cool and moist of center. Perceived to have thinner bodily fluids than men, and greater quantities of them – hence their ability to lactate and their need to menstruate – they are considered to be relatively calm-headed and can sometimes seem to be a little remote. Whether male or female, these doctors assuredly note, people naturally become humorally cooler in their old age. There are many indicative signs of this – not least of which is their need to wear warmer clothes, and their tendency to be adversely affected by cold weather in the winter. For this reason it is important that seniors should not consume certain foods and drinks that will exacerbate the problem and leave them feeling unwell. If an aged person, or indeed anyone, is cooler and moister than necessary, he or she is said to be phlegmatic. This condition can induce a whole range of maladies, not least of which is mental illness due to excess fluids affecting the brain. Deteriorating health in this case can be prevented, and even reversed, by cooking with well-chosen ingredients which, as we shall see, include substances such as cloves, ginger or nutmeg that are humorally hot and dry.

The body can also be overly warm and moist. This means that

it is too blood-rich which makes the patient "sanguine." While some people may consider the plump, ruddy-faced, overly cheerful characteristics of sanguinity agreeable, to others they are undoubtedly irritating; but Renaissance doctors understood that there was a more serious side to this condition. High blood pressure, then as now, was a problem – even if "pressure" was not the term used. A way to combat this potentially dangerous problem is to prepare meals with humorally cool, drying ingredients such as lemon, vinegar or some of the other foods discussed later. Conversely if a person possesses too much black bile, or the wrong kind of this melancholic humor, and is therefore overly cool and dry, he or she requires immediate dietary adjustment of the sort that I will reveal later.

It cannot be overstated that one size certainly does not fit all when it comes to humoral medicine, for the system is inherently individualistic. We have seen that doctors considered laboring men to be on the hot and dry side of center. This requires them to consume specific foods and beverages to prevent illness from occurring and to work effectively. Less active people such as those who sit behind a desk for much of the day, on the other hand, are understood to be closer to midpoint; therefore their bodily requirements are different. Under the humoral system, a more leisurely or studious lifestyle requires the eating of lighter foods that are also relatively low in moisture, coolness and viscosity. The last thing a scholar needs is an excessively phlegm-inducing diet with the resulting impairment to reason and memory.

But whether people work hard for a living or are relatively inactive, medical experts of old knew that humoral complexions and bodily requirements are subject also to climatic conditions. They also knew perfectly well that foods acquire their properties from the environment that surrounds them. Thus, as the body is at one with its natural surroundings, locally produced foods are considered to be the most healthful ones – transferring their humoral properties to the people eating them. To our knowledgeable ancestors this meant that people could safely eat both indigenous plants or animals and those that had been introduced to the region, and had become acclimatized to a particular area over a long period of time. For this reason, olives, dates, figs, citrus fruits, tomatoes and chilies are considered ideal for people living in the Mediterranean basin, the Middle East, and the region described in modern times as the southern United States. For Northern Europeans, and for those living in other cooler places such as Canada, Maine, New Hampshire and New York, temperate and cool-loving plants can just as effectively be used to preserve good health.

Although foreign foods were increasingly used to cure and prevent sicknesses and other bodily disorders in the sixteenth and seventeenth centuries, it was well known that enough plants grew locally to cater for each and every medical requirement. In 1564 physician Philip Moore wrote a small book that was directed specifically at a broad, non-specialist English readership. Adhering to the time-honored, methodical and precise theory and practice of Galenic medicine, he noted that people living in the English climate could maintain and improve their health by choosing the correct diet. This entailed counterbalancing ill humors by eating foods with opposing properties. In suggesting that English people avail themselves of medicines made from plants that readily grow in the English environment, rather than from imported ones better suited to Europeans and Asians, he saw a clear benefit in them propagating their own regional fruits and herbs.

Renaissance physicians knew that both regional difference and the annual weather cycle were factors that required adjustment in diet and healthcare, for Hippocrates himself had written "we must attribute something also to custom, age, season, and region" (*Aphorismes*, Book 1, Aphorism 17, edited by J. van Heurne in 1655). Doctors in England, for example, correctly noted that the chilly, damp winters in their country were bad enough; for this reason they suggest leaving certain phlegm-producing foods alone in order to prevent the onset of winter illnesses, and they argue instead for the eating of "drying" foodstuffs. Drawing on the works of Hippocrates and Galen, the Oxford-educated physician from Somerset, Thomas Cogan, notes this in his 1584 book *The Haven of Health* when he says that adjusting one's diet in the correct manner during the winter months has the effect of shifting one's humoral balance back to the center. In this case he is talking about the benefit of using garlic as an ingredient in meals, but as we will see, some of the driest foodstuffs (in the humoral sense of the word) are liquids. Conversely some dry foods, like granulated sugar, are humorally moist. The change to winter conditions is not a problem specific to cool countries, for it was understood by Renaissance doctors that even in relatively warm regions one is best advised to adjust one's diet depending on the time of the year.

So what are foreign visitors or immigrants to do in order to protect their health when they travel to hotter or colder countries? Galenic advice is clear. Newcomers are affected by their new environment, eventually taking on the characteristics of people who have lived there for a long time. This means that people should closely monitor changes in their humoral complexions and adjust their food intake and medicines according to individual needs. One may see a clear benefit in avoiding rapid changes in diet that can discompose humoral balance, thereby causing illness, and instead assimilate foreign foods gradually. Doctors practicing humoral medicine under-stood this, and they advised caution with regard to stepping out of custom by eating strange foods, or foods that were inappro-priate to the consumer's age, gender and lifestyle.

If medical knowledge of ancient times was readopted by Renaissance physicians, then the validity of this wisdom was also called into question by some humanist thinkers. One was the Swiss physician and alchemist Philip von Hohenheim. Known as Paracelsus, he attributed illnesses to external influences that are treatable by taking medicines made from chemicals and minerals. Although he published several works in the early 1500s, his theories did not gain much support until the mid-1600s. By this time new ideas about the body and its requirements were overtaking even those forwarded by Paracelsus, and anatomical theories continued to develop over the next century. In the face of new ideas, however, traditionalists were skeptical about using chemicals. From experience they had good reason to believe that their health had been maintained effectively by eating the right foods and supplementing this by taking organic medicines. Understanding their own peculiar bodily requirements in humoral terms, many ordinary people, and many doctors, stuck to their beliefs. For example, antiquarian Thomas Baker, who wrote *Reflections upon learning*, was singularly unimpressed with "advancements" in medical science – including the use of chemicals. In 1700, warmly recollecting the golden age of Galenic and Hippocratic medicine that recognized the human body is at one with its natural environment (and should be treated accordingly), he wrote this:

Chemists have appear'd with so much ostentation, and with such contempt of the Arabians and Galen, that we have been made to expect wonders from their performances. Paracelsus, who would be thought the head of a sect, has treated the Galenists so rudely, as if they were the most ignorant men in the world, and had little skill beyond a plaster or a purge.

New procedures and medicines may have worked; but whether or not chemical and mineral medicines were introduced as an attempt to justify the often exorbitant prices for drugs (which can be seen in apothecary D. Gordon's drug price index of 1639), many medical experts and the general public remained absolutely convinced that traditional humoral cures work at least just as well. When one reads medical books published in the late eighteenth and early nineteenth centuries it becomes obvious that natural ingredients with specific humoral properties were still being advocated by doctors to cure illnesses. These include medical works written by, or on behalf of, Guy's Hospital, London (1798), Dr Samuel Tissot (1795), Dr Lewis Robinson (1785), Dr William Buchan (1797) and Dr John Ball (1762). Indeed it will come as no surprise either to herbalists or to proponents of other "alternative" medicines to find humoral cures being advocated and used in the twentieth century and beyond. Looking at the list of cures attributable to lemon vinegar in recent marketing by NU Lifestyle (http://nulifestyle.com/fruit-vinegar/lemon-vinegar/), and to the properties of lemon oil listed by Only Foods (http://www.onlyfoods.net/lemon-oil.html), for example, one can see they are based squarely on humoral medicine – as advocated and practiced by the very same Renaissance doctors to whom I refer throughout these pages.

Chapter Two

Recognizing Your Own Bodily Imbalance

There are many centuries-old diaries and commonplace books (notebooks containing medical and culinary recipes kept usually by household mistresses) that not only describe how to make and take humoral medicines, but also testify to their effectiveness. These recipes, some of which are reproduced later in this book, have been used in bygone days both to prevent and cure an astonishingly wide range of conditions. Preventing illnesses from occurring, however, is undoubtedly a better course of action than rectifying them; as an old proverb notes, it is better to erect a strong fence at the top of a cliff than to park an ambulance at the bottom of it. But however humoral medicine is used, it is dependent upon the user being able to recognize imbalance. This chapter explains how to identify the sort of imbalances that can either give rise to illnesses or can limit the body's ability to deal with them.

By consulting medical guidebooks and training manuals written when humoral medicine was mainstream we get an insight into the way learned physicians thought. We can see how they diagnosed their patients' conditions and understand the processes upon which recovery was based. There are many examples, but one particularly revealing guidebook was written by Knight of the Realm Sir Thomas Elyot. It is called *The castell of helth…wherby euery manne may knowe the state of his owne body*, and was first published in 1536. It proved to be so interesting and useful that it was republished 13 times over the next 74 years.

In this book Elyot notes that if one is sanguine to a dangerous degree one is likely to have a ruddy complexion, be overweight or fleshy and be immoderately jovial. A well-trained doctor would recognize other symptoms, however: the veins and arteries might be large; patients might display a tendency to oversleep; they may dream of pleasant but strange things; the pulse would be strong; the duration of any anger displayed by patients would be short; meals would be digested without any difficulty; and sanguines might bleed easily, have reddish urine, and sweat abundantly. In addition, the senses and wit might be slow; the head might be aching and seem heavy; and the nose could be clogged up. A sanguine person might also display a tendency towards lechery.

What does all this mean, and why might it be important to know these things? A combination of these signs might lead a doctor to suspect that the patient has too much of the blood humor relative to other humors. Taken at face value this might not seem to be particularly problematic. However, "sanguynes," according to the oft-published book *The Regimen of Life*, which was originally written by the medical writer Jean Goeurot in the mid-sixteenth century, are more likely to pick up infections than other people – particularly in the hot summer months. Thus, diseases and infections brought about by the toxins produced when rapid bacterial growth is assisted by warm conditions can be quite harmful to those with this type of complexion. Many physicians like Robert Boyle (*Of the reconcileableness of specifick medicines*, 1685), for example, were also convinced that hemor-rhaging – particularly of the nose and eyes – is more likely to occur in those with a sanguine constitution. By adopting an appropriate diet and lifestyle choices, and using medicines made from well-chosen locally produced ingredients, it is possible to prevent this potentially dangerous complexion and its inherent medical conditions from occurring, and to rectify the problems once they become apparent.

A phlegmatic constitution, like sanguinity, also depends on the body having excess moisture; but unlike a sanguine body it is cold. If one is too phlegmatic, Elyot noted that the signs would be these: The patient might have soft tissue because of the body's moisture level; veins and arteries might be smaller than normal; the person's hearing might be sharper than usual; the complexion is likely to be light in color; and the patient might feel sleepy, but ironically will actually get little in the way of restful sleep. Phlegmatics may dream of water or water-related objects, entities and ideas – such as fish, fishing or riverbanks; and their digestion may be weak. In addition, overly cold, moist people might be slow when they are moving about; they might display impaired mental faculties; there would be a tendency to exhibit timidity; their urine might be paler than one would normally expect, and their spittle is likely to be white and thick and, like nasal mucus, will be present in abundance.

Why might these symptoms be important to recognize? A combination of some of them may well indicate that the patient is indeed phlegmatic; a complexion that is brought about either by having too much of this humor or by having some of it corrupted by other humors. It is said that a phlegmatic constitution is unhealthy in a number of ways, and can induce certain mental and physical issues. It should be noted also that having too much phlegm, or the wrong type of phlegm – often engendered by eating the wrong foods, or the right foods at the wrong time – is particularly problematic to people who are exposed to cool, damp conditions such as those found in Britain in the winter. Some of the phlegmatic issues identified by doctors show that an overabundance of this humor makes the body susceptible to catching a cold, and that coughs and other respiratory problems are engendered by this excessively moist humor traveling through the trachea, bronchi and lungs. Furthermore, the cold and moisture associated with phlegm-producing foods and drinks can potentially affect the mental faculty in a negative way. Humoral dampness is thought to disturb brain patterns and can sometimes impair reason and memory.

A choleric temperament is opposite to a phlegmatic one. It is the result of a humoral imbalance in which either too much yellow bile or corrupted choler is present in the body. The constitution of a choleric person is marked by its heat and dryness which can cause both minor and severe health problems. So how can someone tell if they are overly choleric? In line with the views of physicians, Elyot notes that the bodies of overly hot and dry people might be thin, even if they are well fed; the color of their hair is likely to be black, red or auburn; and although a choleric child might have a good head of hair, as an adult they might be prone to early baldness. They might also be argumentative, cranky and easily angered. A doctor, however, would recognize other symptoms when examining patients: they might be costive; the skin might be red or sallow; they might get little sleep, and dream of heat-related topics or aggression; there could be a tendency towards heat sensitivity; the pulse could be fast and strong; the voice could be sharp; the patient could be quick-witted and watchful; the urine might be clear but highly colored, and there will be little or nothing in the way of excess fluids in the head.

A combination of a number of these symptoms would reveal a humoral imbalance that medical texts inform us could lead to fevers and various forms of blood and bodily infections. It is thought also that an overly choleric temperament can cause infections to spread, particularly around wounded areas. Even the French physician Joseph Du Chesne, who bought into the ideas of alchemist Paracelsus and swallowed them whole, conceded to the existence of yellow choler in his work called *A breefe aunswere of Iosephus Quercetanus Armeniacus*. In discussing the benefits of iron, this doctor noted that an abundance of choler can also result in colic and dysentery. As noted above, a choleric disposition is associated with aggression and short temper, and it is believed that eating humorally hot, dry foods when one is already choleric can cause pyrosis – burning sensations in the stomach and chest. On the plus side, a choleric person will be unlikely to suffer from dull or impaired thinking. The trick, we are told, is to get the balance right. Depending on one's illness, combined with gender, age, lifestyle and personal temperament, this can be achieved by adopting a carefully chosen diet and/or medication.

A melancholic disposition is the result of an overabundance of black bile (or black choler) relative to the other humors, or a result of the body's black bile having been tainted by other humors – usually through disease or eating inappropriate foods. Like choler, black bile characteristically is dry; but it differs in that it is cold. The symptoms of an excessively cold and dry person are typically quietness, an unwillingness to converse on a more-than-necessary basis, and despondency to the point that the patient who suffers from a lack of confidence feels somewhat dejected. In addition, the head will sometimes feel cold. There are, however, other signs that might lead a doctor to suspect that the dangerous and potentially life-threatening condition of melancholy is present. The patient may be thin and have skin that is relatively hard and either duskish or white (melancholy is opposite to sanguinity); there is likely to be a lack of concen-tration evident in adults, but this may not be noticeable in children; the veins and arteries of the patient might be impercep-tible; and the pulse typically is faint. Furthermore the urine is likely to be colorless and thin; the patient is seldom seen to laugh; the person might appear to be timid, fearful and watchful; once roused, the anger will be slow to abate; and the digestion of food might be slow and partial.

Elyot and his contemporary physicians note that a melan-cholic person is prone to picking up infections; this is probably because the body's resistance to disease is at a low ebb. He notes also that anyone so inflicted is likely to show signs of premature aging, as the worrying that is associated with a melancholic nature, then as now, does nothing for one's mental health and physical appearance. This sixteenth-century concern is brought into sharper focus these days, as marketing advertisements reflect an apparent twenty-first-century obsession for projecting an image of youthfulness. Combating the effects of having excessive levels of black choler in the body avoids perturbations of the mind that can lower resistance to infection and, as surgeon Hieronymus Brunschwig notes in *Buch der cirurgia*, published in 1525, avoids having bad dreams and aids restful sleep. Galen himself observed that diseases affecting the skin can be fought by correcting a melancholic complexion, and distiller John Hester in his 1594 book *The pearle of practise* agrees with this. Other medical experts, including women's writer John Partridge (*The Treasurie of Commodious Conceits*, 1591), are absolutely convinced that a melancholic nature is damaging also to internal organs. We will see in Chapter Eight that, somewhat ironically, cold, dry ingredients such as roses and lemons can form the basis of medicines used to cure this problem; these, however, are usually tempered with warm, moist ingredients.

Literacy levels were low during Europe's Renaissance period, and one way of educating people was to impart information in rhyme. Learning mnemonic verses did not just make schooling pleasurable, however; it was also an aid to memory. This worked just as well for students of medicine as it did for students of other subjects. A well-known medical work that came out of Italy's School of Salerno was written in rhyming verse. The author of *Regimen sanitatis Salerni* remains unknown, but it may well have been penned and/or versified by Joannes de Mediolano (John of Milan). In 1541 an English translation of this poem appeared, and over the next century many more similar Galenic and Hippocratic guides to healthful living were published throughout Europe. One of these books, *The English Mans Doctor* by Henrik Rantzau, is based on Mediolano's work. It too was mnemonic to make it easier for the non-specialist to understand, and to facilitate knowledge retention.

Versifying medical instruction may also serve as a useful tool these days; so, in summing up the nature of the humoral body, the last word here should perhaps go to physician William Bullein whose medical treatise *The Government of Health*, published in 1595, helpfully describes the nature of the humoral body in rhyme. The theory that underpins this system, the doctor tells us, came from Hippocrates' book of "windes or blastes." In simple terms humoral medicine entails "putting to the body which it lacketh, or taking from the bodie things superfluous." Bullein cautions that humorism is more complex than this, however, and he notes that "although our life be short, yet the art of phisick is long, because great numbers of things be in it, and requireth much study, labour and practise."

A good place to start, according to the eminent doctor, is to memorize the nature of the four basic complexions. This is the key that will open the treasure chest of lost humoral secrets with which we can "put right that which is wrong:"

The bodies where heat and moysture dwel,
Be sanguine folkes as Galen tell,
With visage faire and cheekes rose ruddy:
The sleep is much and dreames be bluddy.
Pulse great and full, with digestion fine,
Pleasantly concocting flesh and wine,
Excrements aboundant, with anger short,
Laughing very much and finding sport,
Urine grosse, with colour red:
Pleasant folkes at boord and bed.

Where cold with moisture prevaileth much,
Flegmatike folks be alwaies such,
Fatnes, softnes, haire plaine and right,
Narrow veines and colour white,
Dull of wit, no heart, too bold,
Pulse very slow, disgestion cold,

Sleeping over much, urine grosse and pale,
Spittle white and thicke, thus ends the tale.

Choler is hot and drie as fire,
Leannesse of lims and puffed with ire,
Costive bellies, with lite sleepe,
Dreames of fier, or wounds deepe.
Sallowe coloured, or tawnie red,
Feeding on salt meats, and crustes of bread,
Voice sharpe, and quickenes of wit,
Urine yellow and saltnes of spit,
Pulses swift, and verie strong,
Cruell countenance, not anger long.

Melancholy is cold, and very drie,
As here in rime the signes will trie,
Haire plaine, and verie thin,
A leane wretch with hardnes of skin.
Colour whitelie, or like to lead,
Much watch, and dreames of dread,
And stiffe in folish fantasie,
Disgestion slowe, and long angrie.
Fearefull of minde, with watrie spittle,
Seldome laughing, and pulse little,
Urine waterie, and verie thin,
The colde earth to him is kin.

Part II – Long Term Healthfulness

Chapter Three

Fresh Fruits

The rationale upon which the Galenic system is based makes it clear that it is not just the body that contains the four vital humors; it is all organic matter. As humoral characteristics of foods are assimilated by the body, it naturally follows that appropriate food intake is central to healthful living – be it in the form of meals or medicine. Thus, once the current humoral makeup of someone has been established, a diet for maintaining or re-establishing good health can be selected. In Chapter Eight we will be looking at making lotions and potions for relieving or curing a range of medical conditions, and it will be seen that the base ingredients in many of these are either fruits or herbs that possess specific properties. For this reason, and for the fact that this genre of food is usually suitable for vegetarians, vegans and meat eaters alike, I discuss the properties of these foods in this and the next chapter.

"An apple a day keeps the doctor away" according to a popular rhyme. This advice has become more relevant since the campaign to get us to eat at least "five a day" was launched. But crucially, helping to keep the doctor away depends to some extent on the variety of apple being eaten, how it has been prepared, and on the humoral complexion of its consumer.

In general terms fruits, herbs and vegetables in their raw state are often on the cool and moist sides of midpoint, but it is important to realize that this really is a generalization. Humoral characteristics, and therefore nutritional value, depend on many factors. Cooking moderates coolness and moistness, and boiling these foods in water can sometimes, perhaps ironically, reduce the amount of humoral moisture in them. Similarly, processing these foods by adding various edible substances in the cooking process alters their humoral makeup. The addition of spices, for example, may render a cold, moist fruit suitable for a phlegmatic person – even in cool, damp climatic conditions. As the body is at one with nature, affected by environmental conditions and the foods it absorbs, it should not surprise my readers to learn that fruits, herbs and vegetables – like all other foods – are also affected by conditions that surround them. This brings another variable into the equation. A fruit or herb growing on a mountainside will be dryer than one growing near a riverbank or at the edge of marshland; similarly, as Dr Thomas Moffett insightfully notes in his book *Healths Improvement*, an apple growing on the south side of a hill will be humorally warmer than one taken from a tree on the north-facing slope (in the northern hemisphere). Humoral characteristics of plants and fruits also depend on the particular variety. This is not as difficult to determine as one might suppose. Generally, a sweet-tasting apple, cherry or orange, for example, will be humorally "warmer" than a sour one; but, in the words of past dietary experts, not necessarily as nutritious.

On a cold, wet winter's day would a doctor's advice not to eat phlegm-producing fruits like fresh apricots be applicable to everyone, or just to his or her patient? Unlike some well-known dietary advice these days that apparently implies we all have the same nutritional requirements, and that we should eat more fruit and less sugar – seemingly regardless of an individual's medical condition – humorism recognizes, indeed insists, that our needs are individualistic. As Robert Croft notes in his book *Paradise within us*, a work that considers the connection between state of mind and physical health,

forasmuch as neither the matter of Diet nor the quantity thereof…ought to be the same in all sorts of people, but very different according to the diversity of Ages, Complexions,

Constitutions, and the like. It is therefore good that every man be well skilled in the Temperament of his body and mind, that he may be a Rule unto himselfe in that which is best for him.

Thus, advice that is appropriate to a sedentary female office worker in her fifties is different from that which is appropriate to a heat-generating male manual laborer in his late teens. As such, the latter (and possibly both in the summer) might benefit from eating a regulated quantity of cool, moist foods – including fruits like apricots or melons.

Let us now look at the humoral characteristics and medical properties of specific types of the more common fruits in turn. The following characteristics are defined by those whose professional reputations depended on getting it right – physicians of the early modern period such as Dr Henry Butts, Dr Andrew Boorde, Dr William Bullein, Dr James Hart and Dr Thomas Moffett.

Apples

Humoral property:
Sweet varieties are warm in the first degree and temperately moist. Sour varieties are cool and dry.

Positives:
These comfort the heart, quench thirst, dry up phlegm, and relieve a cough. Apples are particularly beneficial to youths and others who have strong stomachs and a choleric temperament.

Negatives:
This fruit can offend weak stomachs, especially when they are eaten raw; eating too many apples may also upset the system. This is because they are very cold and "windy" and hard to digest. They can corrupt the humors and are harmful to phlegmatics.

Advice:
The sweetest varieties are the most nutritious, and they are best when fully ripe. They are most beneficial when roasted, baked or stewed with something humorally warm like pepper, sugar or honey. Ideally apples are eaten in the autumn and spring.

Apricots

Humoral property:
Cold and moist in the second degree.

Positives:
Apricots quench the thirst and dampen the humors in the stomach. The stone of the fruit can kill worms in the body. This fruit is especially beneficial to young people, to those who have a choleric or sanguine temperament, and to those who have strong stomachs.

Negatives:
Because they putrefy other foods already lying in the stomach, they should be eaten *before* other foods. Apricot juices thin the blood, and may be harmful to old people and phlegmatics.

Advice:
The ripest sorts with the deepest color are most beneficial. The stone should be fully ripe and come easily away from the flesh. Apricots are best eaten at the end of May or the beginning of June, especially just before well-seasoned or spiced foods, hard cheese or old wine.

Cherries

Humoral property:
Cold in the first degree, moist in the first or second degree.

Positives:
Cherries are best eaten on an empty stomach, with other foods eaten after them. This is because they prepare the system for digestion. They quench the thirst, cool and moisten the body when consumed in the summer, and stimulate an appetite. They are particularly beneficial in hot weather – especially for youths and cholerics.

Negatives:
They pass through the body quickly, offering little in the way of nourishment. Sweet ones can corrupt the humors in other foods if they are eaten after a meal, but sour ones may be eaten in moderation after a meal. Eating too many can bloat the stomach. Cherries can hurt the aged and very phlegmatic people.

Advice:
The sharpest varieties are more wholesome than the sweet ones, especially those with hard flesh and juice that stains blood red. Eat them when they are freshly picked, but make sure they are completely ripe.

Dates (fresh)

Humoral property:
Hot in the second degree, moist in the first. Green ones are cooler.

Positives:
Although hard to digest, dates are nutritious. Good in moderation in all seasons, and for all ages and constitutions. Although they convert rapidly to choler they do not corrupt other humors. They are nutritious, good for cholerics, they loosen the belly, and they relieve the symptoms of a cough.

Negatives:
Too many can cause dental problems. Dates, which are not good

for the heads of hot people, can induce headaches; they can also cause stomach ache and obstruct the liver and spleen. Eat only a few at most at any one sitting.

Advice:
Sweet and fully ripe dates are the most beneficial. Ideally they should be cooked, but if they are to be eaten raw they should be sprinkled with sugar.

Figs

Humoral property:
Hot in the first degree, moist in the second. Old figs are dryer.

Positives:
Figs are more nourishing than many other fruits. They help to remove gravel and kidney stones, and are good for resisting infections of the blood. Being rapidly digested, the goodness quickly passes to all parts of the body. They quench the thirst and clean out the system. Figs are always in season, but are best in the autumn. They are good for most people and for all constitutions.

Negatives:
When eaten in immoderate quantities they engender crude humors that can cause illnesses to occur – especially colic. They can irritate the liver and spleen. Dates are not particularly good for old folk.

Advice:
White, fully ripe, tender-skinned figs are the most beneficial, red ones are second, and black ones are the least beneficial. They are best eaten with oranges, pomegranates, tart foods, or those pickled in vinegar.

Grapes

Humoral property:
Hot in the first degree, moist in the second.

Positives:
Grapes are best in the spring and autumn, and are good for all but old folk. Although they pass quickly through the system, they nourish and warm the body. They are a fat-producing fruit; they cool the body; they fight inflammation of the liver; and they stimulate urine production.

Negatives:
Grapes cause thirst rather than quench it; they can sometimes cause flatulence and, when eaten in immoderate quantities, they can cause cramps in the stomach. This fruit may also inflame and block the spleen, and can increase defluxions in old folk. Freshly picked grapes are "windy."

Advice:
Fully ripe, thin-skinned grapes are the most beneficial. The white varieties are better for the body than the red varieties. They are at their most efficacious after having been hung up in the sun for two or three days. Eat these moderately just before salt or sour foods rather than after them.

Lemons

Humoral property:
The flesh is cold and dry in the second degree. The rind is warmer and the seeds are hot.

Positives:
The juice is good for promoting appetite. It cuts through and breaks down gross humors, and it is exceptionally useful for fighting infections and fevers. It also helps to dissolve the stone

and cure skin blemishes. Lemon juice and syrup are often the base ingredients in many medicines, as are dried peel and crushed seeds. In a culinary context use moderately, especially with the rind wherever possible.

Negatives:
The lemon does not nourish at all, and it may cool the stomach excessively. It can cause colic and leanness, and, on its own, it can produce melancholic humors. Lemon is unsuitable for the aged, for melancholics, and for people with cold stomachs – such as phlegmatics. This fruit is only suitable for hot weather eating, for youths and for those with choleric or sanguine temperaments.

Advice:
Those with a strong lemon odor are best. Choose those that are a rich yellow color and, ideally, those that were picked a couple of days ago.

Melons

Humoral property:
Cold in the second degree, moist in the third.

Positives:
The melon is useful for cooling the body, particularly in the summer, and for quenching the thirst. It also stimulates the appetite of those who are feeling off-color, it cleanses the humors, and it promotes the production of urine. Eating melon regularly can help to prevent the formation of kidney stones. This fruit is most beneficial to young people and others with hot blood.

Negatives:
Melon nourishes little. It passes through the body quickly and corrupts the humors in foods already lying in the stomach – be

they phlegm or choler. This leaves the body susceptible to illnesses. This fruit can cause flatulence and stomach ache in people with delicate constitutions. The melon should not be eaten by those who suffer from colic, or by splenetic, aged, phlegmatic, or melancholic people.

Advice:
The most flavorsome ones, preferably new and fully ripe, are the best. Eat them with hard cheese, or salt or sour foods, or sharp wine.

Mulberries

Humoral property:
Ripe mulberries are hot and moist in the second degree. Unripe ones are cold and dry.

Positives:
Eating this fruit can remedy a sore throat. It quenches the thirst and can make the body supple. It promotes the appetite and dispels excess choler. Mulberries are best eaten in hot weather, especially by young people and cholerics. Unripe ones may be eaten by sanguines. Mulberry syrup is good for sore throats and is thought by some to help in preventing gout from occurring.

Negatives:
Eating many mulberries may result in stomach upsets and "wind." They should be eaten *before* meals to prevent humoral corruption.

Advice:
The best mulberries are those that are black, plump and fully ripe, and picked in the early morning. Clean them by washing them in wine, and eat sour foods after them.

Olives

Humoral property:
Salty olives are hot and dry in the second degree; the rest are temperate, but are somewhat astringent.

Positives:
Green olives clear the stomach of phlegm, and excel at promoting a healthy appetite. They are also strengthening when eaten during cold weather. Suitable for any constitution.

Negatives:
They are not particularly nutritious. They can inhibit restfulness and can cause headache, especially the salted ones when too many are eaten. Fully ripe olives weaken the stomach and engender gross humors.

Advice:
Green olives are best, especially Italian ones. Eat those that have been steeped in vinegar, rather than salt, to increase appetite, or eat them with other foods in the middle of a meal.

Oranges

Humoral property:
Sweet oranges are more or less neutral; sour ones are cold in the first degree and moist in the second; ones in between are cold and temperately dry. The seeds are humorally hot.

Positives:
The sweet varieties open obstructions, and are good for people suffering from melancholy, and for old folk; they therefore make useful medicines. The middle sort are good for combating fevers and promoting appetite. Sour oranges are useful in hot weather – especially for youths, cholerics and sanguines. A preserve made with orange peel is good for the stomach.

Negatives:

The very sweet varieties are too humorally hot for most people. The sour ones, although best used as a cooking ingredient, are too cool to be eaten on their own, and they can bring on stomach ache, bind the belly, and induce a bloated feeling. They can constrain the breast and arteries. It is best, therefore, to eat very few of them without first moderating them with warming sugar or spices.

Advice:

Large, fully ripe oranges are best – especially those that are neither too sweet nor too sour.

Peaches

Humoral property:

Cold in the first degree, moist in the second. The stones are hot and dry.

Positives:

Good for the heart, peaches freshen the breath by killing odors. This fruit is beneficial to young people and others with choleric or sanguine temperaments.

Negatives:

The humors they introduce to the body are subject to corruption. As such, peaches should be eaten on an empty stomach with a glass of good-quality, fragrant wine. They cause flatulence, and are unsuitable for old folk, phlegmatics, and people with weak stomachs.

Advice:

They should be fully ripe and have a sunset color, a sweet smell and a fresh taste. They should be cooked in wine rather than in water; otherwise they should be roasted. The stone of the peach, if eaten with the raw flesh of the fruit, will temper the humors.

Pears

Humoral property:
Cold in the first degree, dry in the second.

Positives:
This fruit is useful for settling an upset stomach, and it improves the appetite. It is good for removing excess phlegm from the system, and it relieves costiveness.

Negatives:
Similar to the apple; but the pear differs in that it has more superfluous phlegm-producing moisture and it is less durable. The pear is unsuitable for people who suffer from colic or rheumatism, and it should be avoided by the aged. It causes flatulence and may cool the blood excessively.

Advice:
The sweet, dessert varieties are the most beneficial to health. Make sure they are completely ripe. They are best eaten *after* a meal, with good wine and sugar, in the autumn and winter.

Plums

Humoral property:
Cold in the first or second degree, moist in the third or fourth degree.

Positives:
Their coolness and moisture combats any excess of choler in the system – moderating heat and freshening and moistening the body. Plums are good for quenching thirst, promoting appetite, and relieving burning fevers. They are an ideal food for youths, cholerics and sanguines – especially in hot weather.

Negatives:
They loosen and weaken the stomach, they offer very little in the way of nourishment, and they produce watery humors. For this reason, they should be avoided by phlegmatic people, old folk, and those susceptible to colic.

Advice:
Fully ripe, tender and sweet plums that have been picked early in the morning are the most beneficial to health. These should be eaten only on an empty stomach, and, unless being taken medicinally, should be moderated with rose syrup or salted foods. Less ripe plums should be boiled or preserved to correct their crudities.

Pomegranates

Humoral property:
Sweet varieties are warm and moist, and the sour ones are cold and moist.

Positives:
Sweet pomegranates are good during the summer for people of all complexions – providing they are not ill. They strengthen the stomach and the chest by loosening phlegmatic humors, and they relieve coughing. Sour ones are good for the liver, and these are better for cooling fevers suffered by cholerics and young people.

Negatives:
Sweet ones cause flatulence and can also bind the stomach. Sour ones can hurt the teeth and gums. These are unsuitable for aged people, but sweet ones are beneficial to older folk in the winter.

Advice:
Large, fully ripe, sweet pomegranates that are full of juice are the most efficacious. Choose pomegranates from which the skin can

easily be removed.

Strawberries

Humoral property:
Cold and dry in the first degree.

Positives:
Strawberries temper the heat of the blood and lessen any excess of choler. They cool the liver, quench thirst, promote the production of urine, and increase appetite. This fruit is particularly efficacious in hot weather for young people, cholerics and sanguines. The leaves and roots are used in making medicines, and the flesh of the fruit fights fevers and inflammations. Distilled strawberry water cleans the kidneys and urinary passages and flushes out ill humors.

Negatives:
Cultivated strawberries are unsuitable for phlegmatics on account of their coolness, and should not be eaten by people with inflamed sinews or weak stomachs. Wild strawberries should be avoided on account of their sourness that offends the stomach.

Advice:
Those that are red, very ripe and fragrant are the best. Their coldness and dryness can be corrected by eating them with sugar and red wine. Cream on strawberries should be avoided by people with weak constitutions – such as delicate, sedentary women.

The importance of fruit as a nutritious food has been recognized since biblical times, and ever since then it has been appreciated by many in humanity's quest for longevity and good health. This kind of food, Doctor Moffett notes, is commended for three reasons: "antiquity, purity, and sufficiency." As we have seen, different fruits have different humoral characteristics; this means that there is something for everyone, and as long as they are prepared correctly and eaten at the right time they are beneficial to the mind and body. The eminent physician points out that fruits have been successfully grown and eaten to "maintain us in long life" for ages, and that they still are the principal food in some countries of the world. Furthermore, he says, the hands of people who eat fruits are not "polluted with the blood of beasts," and this sort of food can sustain a healthy and long life without the need for "any great dressing." The same applies to herbs and vegetables; and it is to these foods we now turn.

Chapter Four

Herbs and Vegetables

Dietary advice seems to change almost on a weekly basis, with the assumptions of one group of researchers casting doubts on those of another. Long-held beliefs are assuredly cast aside as certain foods or beverages considered indispensable last year are now, according to the latest survey of "x" number of people suffering from "y" disease, supposedly bad for us. Contradictions are everywhere. Despite this, greens, modern nutritionists currently believe, are essential to maintaining good health. The humoral position also recognizes the nutritional medical value of herbs and vegetables, and it always has; but humorism considers finely the different values of every sort, and their suitability for people with diverse complexions.

Eating the animal products discussed in Chapters Six and Seven is not necessary, strictly speaking, to ensure good health. Like the diverse properties attributed to fruits, the medical characteristics of a broad range of herbs and vegetables also show us that there is sufficient difference between them to cater for everyone – regardless of the consumer's health and temperament. In this chapter I discuss the nutritional values of some of the more common greens from the humoral point of view. Again, these characteristics are sourced from the works of eminent medical practitioners whose professional reputations relied on disseminating accurate information:

Artichoke (globe)

Humoral property:
Hot in the second degree, dry in the first.

Positives:

Not only are artichokes tasty, they can be beneficial insofar as they bring humoral heat to the stomach and intestines, they promote the production of urine that flushes away gross humors, and they open obstructions in the digestive system. This prevents blockages from occurring; blockages that can corrupt the humors and attract a variety of illnesses. The artichoke is an ideal winter vegetable for phlegmatics.

Negatives:

This vegetable is slightly flatulent. Eating it raw can cause headache, and too much cooked artichoke can induce stomach ache. It should be avoided by young people in the summer.

Advice:

The artichoke is best eaten after having been boiled in water until thoroughly tender, along with meat or other vegetables.

Asparagus

Humoral property:

Hot in the first degree, temperately moist.

Positives:

Like the artichoke, asparagus opens up any obstructions that may be in the digestive system or liver. It also loosens the belly and promotes the production of urine – cleaning the kidneys. This vegetable is a healthful addition to the foodways of people of all ages – to all but those with the most choleric of temperaments. This vegetable is particularly beneficial to aged people, to people with poor eyesight, and to melancholics.

Negatives:

If eaten raw, asparagus can cause sickness. Its natural heat, along with its slight bitterness, increases choler production. This is something that cholerics should be wary of.

Advice:
The tops of freshly grown asparagus, harvested and then cooked and eaten straight away, are the most wholesome part of the plant. It should be boiled in water until it is soft, and tempered with oil, vinegar, pepper and salt.

Beans (green)

Humoral property:
Cold in the first degree, dry in the second.

Positives:
This vegetable facilitates sleep and can build up the body. Beans are particularly beneficial in cold weather, and act as an antidote to sanguinity.

Negatives:
Beans cause flatulence and can dull the senses. Although they aid sleep, this is seldom restful as eating them can induce disturbing dreams. They lie long in the stomach, leaving them susceptible to corruption from any other undigested or partly digested foods. This can lead to stomach upsets.

Advice:
This legume is a good source of nutrition. Young and tender beans are the most efficacious – particularly those without blemishes. Remove the tops and bottoms, and cook them thoroughly with salt and marjoram, or better still with onion, in order to correct their crudities.

Beetroot

Humoral property:
Cold in the first degree, moist in the second.

Positives:
Eating beetroot opens up any obstructions, allowing for the ejection of gross humors, and they admirably loosen the belly. Beets' humoral coolness and moistness is particularly good for moderating choleric temperaments.

Negatives:
Being a little windy, beets can cause stomach upsets, particularly in people who have a phlegmatic constitution.

Advice:
Best used in salads, they should be boiled to remove excess humoral moisture, and then they should be sliced. Add to them drying oil or vinegar. They may safely be eaten with wine and pepper by phlegmatics.

Borage

Humoral property:
Cold and moist in the first degree.

Positives:
This herb purifies the blood, and is particularly useful because it helps to remove corrupted humors. It refreshes the body and uplifts the heart and spirits, especially when added to wine and taken as a tonic. Borage is also said to strengthen the intestinal tract, and it is very good for convalescents. It can be used as a laxative. It is one of the few herbs that is suitable for all ages and complexions, and it can usefully be eaten during any season.

Negatives:
It is not particularly nutritious, and its goodness is absorbed by the body slowly. It can be troublesome to people with sore mouths.

Advice:

The most common sort to be used as a medicine in pastimes is the "bugloss" plant from which the leaves and flowers are used. It can be used in a salad or cooked in meat stew or soup.

Brassica (cabbage, broccoli, sprouts, kale)

Humoral property:

Cold and moist in the first degree. When cooked it is hot in the first degree and dry in the second.

Positives:

Depending on how it is prepared, it can be used either to bind the belly (eating well-cooked leaves, florets or stems) or as a laxative (boiling the juice in a casserole, for example). Leaves soaked in honey can kill worms and cure ulcers, and eating leaves is thought also to help cure gout. Brassica leaves can be used as plasters to help cure infections. Broth made from this vegetable, if eaten on an empty stomach, can help to prevent drunkenness.

Negatives:

Brassicas are not digested very quickly. They may be too cool and moist for people with very phlegmatic constitutions, unless they are corrected with drying ingredients. Being cold and somewhat dryer, cabbage can induce thick, melancholic vapors that sometimes adversely affect the mental faculties and weaken the sight.

Advice:

Young leaves, shoots and buds of freshly harvested, tender plants should be used. Boil them in water, then cook them with meat and drying pepper. Wild plants of the brassica family have similar properties.

Burnet

Humoral property:
Hot and dry in the second degree.

Positives:
This herb is still used widely and appreciated for its advantageous urinary tract properties. It is believed to purge the kidneys and bladder of gross humors, to promote urine, and to dispel stones and gravel. When eaten with wine it comforts the heart.

Negatives:
The goodness of burnet is slow to be assimilated by the body, and the herb itself lies long in the stomach – attracting the production of unwanted crude humors. Although used to treat infectious diseases in past times, its humoral heat and dryness can inflame the liver and blood. Cholerics should be wary of eating burnet.

Advice:
Usually found wild with small serrated and red stems, this usefully warming and drying plant can easily be grown in gardens. Eat raw in salads, but moderate its properties with cooling herbs.

Carrot

Humoral property:
Hot in the second degree, moist in the first.

Positives:
The carrot promotes the production of urine that clears the system of gross, infection-inducing humors. It also opens up obstructions. This root vegetable may be particularly useful for women, as it is thought to aid menstruation and the production of milk. It is more beneficial medically than the parsnip that has similar properties.

Negatives:
The carrot is slowly digested and is therefore susceptible to humoral corruption. It nourishes very little compared to leaf vegetables. It can cause flatulence.

Advice:
The most useful carrots are large, sweet ones with the deepest natural color. Boil them thoroughly and eat them corrected with oil, mustard and coriander. Best in cold weather, carrots are beneficial to all but old folk and phlegmatics.

Chicory

Humoral property:
Cold in the first degree; dry in the second.

Positives:
Its humoral coolness helps to cure an inflamed stomach, and eating this plant opens obstructions in and around the liver. Chicory is a useful addition to the meals of youths and others with hot constitutions – particularly, but not exclusively, in the summer.

Negatives:
It can exacerbate weak stomachs, especially those of melancholics, and it affords the eater very little in the way of nourishment.

Advice:
The blue flowers and the tops of chicory are the most beneficial parts. It can be eaten raw, but it is best boiled and then eaten in salads with vinegar and humorally hot herbs such as mint.

Cucumber

Humoral property:
Cold and moist in the second degree.

Positives:
Technically a fruit, this gourd is best for hot and dry constitutions – especially when eaten in the summer. If eaten in moderate quantities, it is easily digested.

Negatives:
The cucumber affords little if any nourishment, it is "windy," and eating it may harm the digestive systems of old people. It may also harm those with cold stomachs, and people who are phlegmatic. It is thought that eating cucumber too frequently can cause cold, thick humors to accumulate in the veins; this leaves the body susceptible to contracting illnesses.

Advice:
Cucumbers are best harvested and eaten while they are still quite small. To prepare them in a way that partially moderates their crudities, one should slice them and steep them in drying vinegar. They should be eaten with oil, or with hot, drying pepper.

Endive

Humoral property:
Cold in the first degree, moist in the first or second.

Positives:
Endives sharpen the appetite, reduce inflammation and quench the thirst. They also benefit the body by promoting the flow of urine that lessens the buildup of disease-inducing humors. In warm weather, endives are particularly beneficial to youths, cholerics, sanguines, and others with humorally hot stomachs.

Negatives:
Endive, particularly too much of it, is bad for those that suffer from palsy, and for people with cold stomachs. This plant is digested slowly.

Advice:
Tender but not too young, freshly harvested endive is the most beneficial to the body. It should be eaten with mint, rue (herb of grace), or other hot herbs to correct its phlegm-inducing properties.

Fennel

Humoral property:
Hot in the second or third degree, dry in the first.

Positives:
This herb promotes the production and passing of urine, opens obstructions in the body and purges the kidneys of waste. All of this helps to remove corrupt illness-producing humors from the body. It is particularly beneficial to women insofar as it aids menstruation and the production of milk. Fennel is also good for the eyesight. Beneficial at any time, particularly in the winter, this herb is very good for most people – including phlegmatics and old folk.

Negatives:
It can inflame the blood, reducing the quantity of beneficial humors there. Both in its raw and cooked states it is difficult to digest – especially when much of it is eaten. Fennel is not particularly beneficial to young people and cholerics.

Advice:
Newly harvested young fennel is best if it is to be eaten fresh. If it is to be stored and eaten at a later date, it should be mature and

kept in cold water. Eat only small quantities.

Garlic

Humoral property:
Hot in the fourth degree, dry in the third.

Positives:
When served cooked or raw, its extreme humoral heat and dryness acts as a very effective counterbalance to cool, moist foods. Garlic resists poisons and fights infections, it clears the throat, it kills worms, it cleanses the stomach, and it aids the production and flow of urine to remove impurities from the body. Garlic is ideal in cold weather, especially for old people and phlegmatics.

Negatives:
It can cause a dulling of the mental faculties, induce headache, and adversely affect the eyesight. It can also revive old diseases. Garlic should be avoided by pregnant women, and by youths and people with choleric constitutions.

Advice:
Use early garlic (ready between February and April at a latitude of 51 to 54 degrees) raw in salads. For cooking, use later varieties and boil them thoroughly before adding to other foods.

Hops

Humoral property:
Temperately neutral regarding heat, moist in the first degree.

Positives:
A useful herb if one's humors are out of balance, for hops engender good humors and at once help to rectify humoral imbalance. Hops refine and purify the blood and strengthen the

digestive tract. Used as a preservative to lengthen the life of beer, hops are suitable for any age and humoral complexion. They can be consumed safely in any season.

Negatives:
Having a rather bitter taste, hops can be slightly flatulent; and eating too many of them bloats the stomach and causes headache.

Advice:
Use only the fresh, tender buds and shoots. They are best boiled in water and eaten with oil and vinegar to humorally dry them.

Leeks

Humoral property:
Hot in the third degree, dry in the second.

Positives:
The leek is not as hot as garlic, and it has different properties: it promotes urine, aids monthly fluxes in women, and has mild aphrodisiacal powers. Leeks can help to expel gross humors in the form of gases, for they are quite windy. When eaten with honey they can lessen the effects of respiratory tract problems; and when applied as a plaster the leaves can help cure hemorrhoids.

Negatives:
Leeks can generate melancholic humors, and therefore are unsuitable for melancholics. This vegetable can also impair the memory, dim the eyesight, and induce bad dreams or nightmares. Furthermore it can cause stomach ache, and when eaten in inordinate quantities it can generate ulcers in the bladder. The leek makes a better medicine than a source of nourishment.

Advice:
When growing leeks it is advisable to keep the soil well-watered. Harvest them while they are still small and tender in order to limit their humoral dryness. Soak them thoroughly, dress them in oil, and eat them with cool and moist leaves like lettuce or endives.

Lettuce

Humoral property:
Cold and moist in the second degree.

Positives:
Although it affords little nourishment, lettuce is easily digested. This admirable quality means that after a short time there is none of it left in the system to cause, attract or be affected by corrupt humors. It is the best of all salad ingredients. It is thought to increase milk in women, it aids restful sleep, it cleanses the kidneys, and it removes choler-generating heat from the stomach – especially when it is eaten after being sprinkled with humorally cold and dry lemon juice or vinegar. It is especially beneficial to young people, cholerics, and others suffering from excess heat in the stomach.

Negatives:
Lettuce can dim the eyesight and remove natural heat from the body, weakening the stomach and leaving it susceptible to infection. It is thought to cause infertility, to dampen the eater's sex drive, and to make the body sluggish.

Advice:
Best grown in rich soil, the lettuce should be harvested before it reaches its full size. In order to temper the illness-producing phlegmatic properties of this food, it should be cleaned but not washed in cold water. Ideally it should be boiled rather than

served raw, and eaten with humorally hot, dry leaves like mint or rue.

Marjoram

See properties of **Rosemary**.

Mint

Humoral property:
Hot and dry in the second or third degree.

Positives:
Mint is very efficacious to people suffering from cold and weak stomachs, and is an admirable herb for comforting the body and removing fluxes. Mint sharpens the appetite, cleans the kidneys, kills worms, and it helps to burn away phlegmatic humors that would otherwise leave the body susceptible to contracting diseases. Best eaten in cold weather, this herb is ideal for old people and both phlegmatics and melancholics.

Negatives:
Mint can irritate a hot stomach or liver. This herb should be avoided by cholerics.

Advice:
As the stems and old leaves are the hottest, only the young new leaves should be used. Eat mint sparingly in a meal that contains humorally cold herbs.

Onions

Humoral property:
Hot in the third degree, dry in the second.

Positives:
The onion contains humors that are aphrodisiacal and at once

increase fertility. They help to produce milk in women of child-bearing age, they sharpen the appetite, and they warm the bodies of aged people and those with phlegmatic constitutions. Cutting through gross humors, they also promote the passing of urine, open obstructions and combat kidney stones.

Negatives:
If they are eaten in immoderate quantities after having been cooked, or at all in their uncooked state, they can cause headache and introduce bad humors to the blood. They can dull the mental faculties, dim the eyesight, and induce bad dreams. This food is not suitable for cholerics, particularly in the summer.

Advice:
Best grown in well-watered soil, the most beneficial onions are those that are large, round and full of juice. To moderate their humoral heat and dryness they should be sliced and soaked in cold water for a while. Cooking them diminishes their medical attributes, but at the same time it reduces their negative qualities. Eating much onion induces sound sleep.

Parsley

Humoral property:
Hot in the second degree, dry in the first.

Positives:
Parsley is particularly efficient at flushing out the urinary tract; it also opens up obstructions, cleans the liver and kidneys, and aids menstruation. It is easy on the stomach, and its humoral properties allow this herb to resist infection. When cooked it is good for all ages and constitutions at any time of year.

Negatives:
When eaten raw it can inflame the humors, and in large

quantities uncooked parsley can also cause headache and dim the eyesight. As it is digested slowly it can corrupt, or be corrupted by, other foods in the stomach. Those with choleric temperaments should be wary of eating this herb in its uncooked state.

Advice:
Best harvested when the leaves are still young, and before the plant flowers. Eat it only in small quantities with herbs that are humorally cold, or cook it thoroughly and add it to a meal.

Parsnip

Humoral property:
Hot in the second degree, temperately moist.

Positives:
Although this vegetable is humorally hot it offers good nourishment. Even so, it is not as nutritious as the carrot.

Negatives:
It lingers long in the digestive system, which puts at risk other foods lying there, and it is slightly windy.

Advice:
The parsnip is best boiled with the addition of cooling vinegar, and then buttered.

Peas

Humoral property:
Cold in the first degree, temperately moist.

Positives:
Peas are an excellent source of nourishment and they are digested more rapidly than green beans. They clean the breast,

kidneys and bladder, and can help to relieve a cough. Best eaten in warm weather, they are particularly beneficial to physically active people, to youths and to people with a choleric temperament.

Negatives:
Peas should be avoided by phlegmatic people and by those who suffer from flatulence.

Advice:
Small, new tender peas should be selected, as larger ones more easily corrupt the humors. Prepare them with drying ingredients such as salt, pepper, vinegar or citrus juice.

Potato

Humoral property:
Hot in the second degree, moist in the first.

Positives:
The potato is better than root vegetables at strengthening the body, soothing the stomach and expelling urine. It is most beneficial to people with a melancholic nature.

Negatives:
It is slightly windy. Sanguines should be wary of eating too many potatoes or those that are "uncorrected."

Advice:
Early varieties and small ones are the most beneficial to health, and they are best well-boiled and eaten with cooling and drying leaves.

Radish

Humoral property:
Hot in the second degree, dry in the first.

Positives:
The radish makes a good medicine, for it has a cutting quality, and cuts effectively through phlegm. It helps to clear the urinary tract, and, like the juice and flesh of the lemon, it can help to break up and remove stones and gravel. It also cleans the stomach and the throat. Radishes are best eaten in cold weather, and they are particularly beneficial to phlegmatics.

Negatives:
It induces wind, and can cause headache, toothache, dim eyesight and hot-bloodedness. Digestion of the radish is slow. This root is not for people with gout or rheumatism.

Advice:
Thin, tender young radishes are least harmful to cholerics. They are best eaten at the end of a meal.

Rosemary

Humoral property:
Hot and dry in the second degree.

Positives:
Beneficial to most people, rosemary fights cold humors and comforts the brain and heart. Rosemary helps prevent old illnesses from reoccurring, it fights palsy, and it encourages sweating. Taken with pepper and honey it relieves a cough. It is an admirable herb to be consumed in the winter by old or phleg-matic people. Rosemary water, made with the flowers, is a good medicine to combat illnesses brought on by having an excess of melancholic humors.

Negatives:
Choleric people should be careful not to eat too much rosemary –
especially in the summer.

Advice:
Only young, light green leaves should be used. Steep in cold
water, and then serve with humorally cooling leaves.

Sage

Humoral property:
Hot and dry in the second or third degree.

Positives:
Sage can help to treat palsy and quivering of the joints. If eaten at
the onset of a cold it comforts the head and relieves the senses.
This herb sharpens the memory, and it has styptic powers that,
when applied to a wound, help to stop bleeding. It cleans a cold,
moist womb, aids conception, and moderates women's immoderate fluxes. It is beneficial to old people, people with cold
stomachs, and to phlegmatics – especially in the winter and
spring.

Negatives:
It can be troublesome to melancholics by over-drying them, and
it can exacerbate choleric problems by overheating those who
have hot complexions.

Advice:
As is the case with most herbs, the younger leaves taken from the
top of the stem are the most beneficial. Either eat it in salads with
cold, moist leaves such as lettuce, or cook it and eat it with moist
meats or vegetables.

Sorrell

Humoral property:
Cold in the first degree, dry in the second.

Positives:
Sorrell is a very profitable herb from a health point of view. It helps to reduce the effects of having too much of the choler humor – curing fluxes and lessening the likelihood of contracting fevers and infectious diseases. It quenches the thirst and stimulates the appetite. It is good in hot weather, and beneficial to sanguine and choleric people.

Negatives:
It can induce stomach ache and bind the belly. Sorrell can be detrimental to melancholics.

Advice:
Choose only the pure green leaves. Eat it in salads with warming herbs such as mint, or make a green sauce with it.

Spinach

Humoral property:
Cold and moist in the first degree.

Positives:
Spinach strengthens the breast, relieves the symptoms of a cough, and cools inflammations in the chest. It is good for all ages and constitutions, especially for youths and cholerics.

Negatives:
It is somewhat windy, it can irritate the stomach, and it engenders watery humors in cold stomachs.

Advice:
Ideally this vegetable should be fried or steamed (rather than boiled), and then corrected with oil and humorally warm ingredients like raisins.

Tarragon

Humoral property:
Hot and dry in the second degree.

Positives:
This flavorsome herb stimulates the appetite and comforts the head, heart and stomach. It is particularly beneficial to old folk and to phlegmatics.

Negatives:
Tarragon attenuates the blood humor in cholerics, and it can inflame the liver.

Advice:
Only the tenderest leaves should be used. To moderate its humoral heat and dryness it should be eaten sparingly with cooling herbs such as borage, endives or lettuce.

Tomato

Humoral property:
Cold and moist in the second or third degree.

Positives:
Like the cucumber, the tomato is technically a fruit. It is best eaten in warm climates, but is also valuable to people who have hot and dry constitutions – especially when eaten in the summer. The tomato falls under the domination of Venus, and may cause a desire for sexual indulgence.

Negatives:
Tomatoes offer very little nourishment to the body, and the digestion of them is slow and partial. This breeds melancholic humors that can corrupt the blood. Furthermore they are somewhat "windy."

Advice:
As long as they are fully ripe, tomatoes may be eaten in moderation as a salad ingredient along with oil, salt or pepper. However, it is better to roast them, or to sprinkle them with flour and fry them in oil or butter with a little drying pepper and salt. Tomatoes grown in cool countries should be avoided on account of their watery and insipid nature.

The humoral physician Dr Philip Moore, who practiced medicine in the English county of Suffolk, noted that home-produced herbs and vegetables, just like locally grown fruit, had been "founde by long experience to bee moste holsome and profitable against an infinite number of diseases." He considered the practice of having medicines "brought out of India, or from the furthest parte of the worlde" lamentable when locally grown produce admirably did the trick. Moore notes also that since biblical times this type of food has nourished "multitudes of people in diverse ages," and still does in some communities, without recourse to eating animal flesh.

Although people have different humoral complexions, and therefore different health requirements, we have seen that there is a wide enough range of herbs and vegetables available to maintain and restore good health, and at once enjoy a varied and interesting diet. As is the case for tarragon and some of the other herbs discussed here, humoral heat is usually attributed to exotic spices, dried fruits and condiments. These substances that in a culinary sense alter the taste, texture and fragrance of foods have, and have had since medieval times, very important medical values. Additives that fall into this category – from pepper and cinnamon to raisins and sugar – are discussed next.

Chapter Five

Spices, Condiments and Dried Fruits

Ever since European merchants and travelers first visited the Far East looking for wealth and material riches, or for knowledge and adventure, spices have had a special role in European and, subsequently, American cooking. But before spices were used in a modern-style culinary sense they became increasingly important as medicines – especially among the well-to-do who could afford to buy expensive luxuries. Why was this? It all revolves around humoral medical thinking. Although medical practitioner Philip Moore was completely underwhelmed by the health benefits of cooking with, or making medicines out of, exotic substances (preferring instead to use locally grown produce), not all doctors agreed. It became obvious to some physicians and dietary experts that the properties many spices exhibit, heat and dryness obtained from their growing environment, are very useful in "correcting" potentially health-damaging meals. Not all "spices" are hot and dry, however. Sugar, which originated in India, and dried fruits like raisins and currants, and honey, are also classified as spices in humoral texts. These humorally warm and moist foods brought the fight against melancholic illnesses to a whole new level. This genre of food includes, of course, condiments like pepper and mustard, but it also includes table salt – a mineral that, perhaps puzzlingly until one considers its properties, was listed in the spice and sauce section of some medical books.

The humoral characteristics of spices like cinnamon, nutmeg and ginger do not lose their potency when added to other foods and drinks. Instead these spices transfer their heat and dryness to them. Thus, a wine so treated can be classified as "dry." I personally know people who can testify that after drinking

Become Your Own Doctor

mulled wine (or glühwein) on a cold winter's evening, they were not only warmed up by it, but were also dried of excess fluids in the head at the same time. Their feet became warmer and nasal discharge was effectively stemmed. Not everyone would benefit from drinking this spice-laden beverage of course. We will recall from Chapters One and Two that our humoral complexions and bodily requirements differ one from the other, and that our personal qualities need to be established in order to get the most out of foods and drinks. Having said that, I will now reveal the humoral characteristics and medical attributes of many of the more commonly used spices, as seen by the distinguished experts mentioned previously.

Cinnamon

Humoral property:
Hot in the third degree, dry in the second.

Positives:
This spice facilitates the passing of urine, which clears the system of gross illness-inducing humors, and it resists poisons and helps to prevent the blood from becoming contaminated. Cinnamon sharpens the mental faculties and strengthens the intestines. Its dryness is beneficial to the eyes, which would otherwise be weakened by eating humorally moist and viscose foods. It is an ideal additive to foods and beverages in cold weather, and it is useful to old people and others with cold and weak stomachs.

Negatives:
If consumed immoderately cinnamon can be damaging to the health of cholerics and people with hot stomachs, especially in hot weather. It can inflame the internal organs and heat the blood.

Advice:
Only the newest fine, thin cinnamon sticks should be used. They should smell sweet, have a sharp taste, and be red in color. Use sparingly when adding this spice to humorally cold or moist foods.

Cloves

Humoral property:
Hot and dry in the third degree.

Positives:
This spice strengthens the organs, especially the stomach, heart and liver. It helps to regulate and correct bodily fluxes, and it is useful for neutralizing bad breath. Cloves aid digestion, help to prevent fainting and infection, and are very beneficial to health during the winter – especially to the aged and to phlegmatics.

Negatives:
Their heat can adversely affect people with hot constitutions like young men and cholerics. This is particularly the case when they are eaten in the summer.

Advice:
Small, young and fresh cloves that are slightly moist and have a piquant aroma are the most beneficial. Add them to milk, or put small quantities of them in humorally moist food when the head and body of the patient contain excess fluids. Using too many is excessively drying, and will impart an unpleasant, bitter taste.

Ginger

Humoral property:
Green ginger is hot in the third degree and moist in the first. Dry ginger is hot in the third degree and dry in the second.

Positives:

Ginger helps to break wind that would otherwise corrupt the humors. It is good for warming cold stomachs, but heats the body more slowly than pepper. It aids digestion, cuts through the worst of the phlegmatic humors, and it sharpens the eyesight. It also sharpens the memory if eaten on an empty stomach in the morning. This spice is best added to foods in the winter, and is particularly efficacious to elderly people and phlegmatics.

Negatives:

This spice can inflame the blood and stomach of cholerics and others with hot constitutions, especially when consumed during hot weather.

Advice:

Use only fresh young roots. They should have a pleasing smell and a sharp taste. Use green ginger mixed with honey to warm old people's stomachs. If using dry ginger, use it only in moderate quantities. Young people should use green ginger.

Honey

Humoral property:
Hot and dry in the second degree.

Positives:

Honey warms up the stomach; it resists putrefaction of the humors, and therefore reduces the chance of becoming ill; and it is valuable in neutralizing costiveness. It is beneficial to the digestive systems of old folk in winter, and to people suffering from rheumatism.

Negatives:

Honey increases the amount of choler in the body, and, if eaten in immoderate quantities, it is believed to inflame the blood. It may exacerbate any problems suffered by those who have hot complexions.

Advice:
Pure, clear honey, light in color, is the best for good health. It should also be new and thick. It is most beneficial when it is eaten with fruit or sour foods, or with rose syrup.

Mace

Humoral property:
Hot in the second degree, dry in the third.

Positives:
This spice is derived from nutmeg, and it has similar positive qualities. It is thought that adding mace to a beverage helps to stop the spitting of blood, and that mace added to food can help combat bloody fluxes. It strengthens the bodies of people with cold, moist constitutions. This spice is good for settling the stomach.

Negatives:
Like most hot and dry spices, this one is not recommended for people whose bodies contain an abundance of choler. This is particularly so during spells of warm weather.

Advice:
It is most useful when taken in small quantities.

Mustard

Humoral property:
Hot in the fourth degree, dry in the second.

Positives:
This makes an excellent sauce for counterbalancing the

moistness and coolness of a variety of foods – such as the fish and the meat of young animals discussed in the next two chapters. It purges the brain of damaging cold, vaporous humors, and cuts through gross illness-inducing humors in the stomach. It can cause sneezing, which usefully expels unwanted humors. Mustard is best eaten in cold weather, and is beneficial to old people, phlegmatics and rheumatics.

Negatives:
Despite its dryness it is not good for the eyesight. Cholerics should be wary of eating mustard – especially in hot weather.

Advice:
Eat this only as a sauce to accompany and rectify cold, moist foods.

Nutmeg

Humoral property:
Hot and dry in the second or third degree.

Positives:
Nutmeg is good for the skin as it removes blemishes, it fights bad breath, and it maintains sharp eyesight. Internally it can help to soothe the spleen and stomach, and it stimulates the passing of urine which rids the body of bad humors. This spice is excellent in winter for old folk and people who suffer from having excessive levels of phlegm in their systems.

Negatives:
As this spice binds the belly, it can hurt those who are constipated. It may be harmful to people with a melancholic character, and to those suffering from hemorrhoids.

Advice:

Choose only young, fresh nutmegs that are quite large and moist, but not green ones. The latter are too young and not very beneficial to health. The color of them should be reddish. Use this spice only occasionally, and in moderation, with a little ginger. It is most efficacious when eaten in the morning.

Pepper

Humoral property:
Hot and dry in the third degree.

Positives:
Pepper helps to aid the digestive process. It stimulates the appetite, helps to breaks wind – ridding the body of gross, vaporous, illness-inducing humors – and it strengthens the stomach. It is effective at heating the sinews and muscles, and it cuts through phlegmatic humors. It also aids urination. Pepper is particularly beneficial in the winter, and is good for the aged, for phlegmatics, and for rheumatics.

Negatives:
Pepper may be harmful to people with hot constitutions, especially when it is eaten in hot weather. It is thought to reduce fertility in men, and can overheat the blood when immoderately used.

Advice:
Only peppercorns that are small, new and free from wrinkles should be chosen. They should be coarsely ground and used moderately in cold weather to counterbalance the phlegmatic properties of cold, moist or viscose meats.

Raisins

Humoral property:
Warm in the first degree, moist in the second.

Positives:
Raisins, especially Spanish ones, stimulate the appetite and provide the body with wholesome nourishment. They are good for fighting stomach disorders, and are good for the liver and respiratory system. They also loosen the belly.

Negatives:
Raisins should be avoided by people with sanguine or choleric constitutions on account of their heat.

Advice:
Choose the large, sweet ones and eat them before meals. Inferior ones are less effective. Useful for moderating the effects of melancholic humors.

Saffron

Humoral property:
Hot in the second degree, dry in the first.

Positives:
Often used as a coloring agent, saffron can help to preserve the intestines and soothe the heart. Like many spices it is thought to stimulate the production and passing of urine, and is thought also to increase sex drive, aid menstruation and hasten childbirth. Some believe it is a good cure for drunkenness, and that it cleans the liver and fights jaundice. Most efficacious in the winter, this spice is a useful addition to the meals of old people, phlegmatics and melancholics.

Negatives:
Taken in immoderate quantities it can make the head feel heavy, it can cause drowsiness, and it diminishes the appetite. Saffron may not be suitable for cholerics.

Advice:
Choose fresh, naturally bright-colored saffron that has a fragrant aroma. In cold weather, a moderate amount of this spice is a good addition to meals that predominantly are cold in the humoral sense of the word.

Salt

Humoral property:
Warm in the first degree, dry in the second.

Positives:
Used in the preparation of many foods, salt is an excellent natural preservative that, through the valuable process of osmosis, works by inhibiting the growth of bacteria. Thought to resist poison, salt cuts through and consumes all corrupt phlegmatic humors. Used sparingly, it may be beneficial in cold weather to phlegmatics and people who have cold stomachs.

Negatives:
Salt can dry the body and blood to a dangerous level, and can result in premature aging of the skin, and in skin blemishes. It is thought to reduce fertility in men. Salt is particularly bad for young people and cholerics.

Advice:
Choose pure white, hard and dry salt for preserving foods. In the absence of a suitable alternative, use very sparingly to correct humorally moist foods.

Sugar

Humoral property:
Warm and moist in the first degree.

Positives:
Like salt, sugar is another excellent preservative that works by inhibiting the growth of bacteria through the process of osmosis. It is thought to clean the body, especially the chest, and to be wholesome for the kidneys. Brown sugar is said to be as nourishing as honey. Good for most constitutions at all times of the year – especially for old folk in the winter.

Negatives:
Sugar can cause thirst, and it readily turns to choler that can be damaging to people with hot constitutions. It can rot the teeth, it can increase blood humors to a level that might attract disease, and it can cause bad breath.

Advice:
Sugar is best with sour or humorally cold, dry foods – such as many fruits.

Vinegar

Humoral property:
Cool in the first degree, dry in the second.

Positives:
In addition to being a preservative, although not as effective as salt, it tempers excessive body heat. It strengthens weak gums and is particularly efficient at breaking and eradicating phlegmatic humors and fighting infections. Vinegar is best used in hot weather, and it is especially beneficial to young people and sanguines.

Negatives:
Taken on an empty stomach it can cause stomach and intestinal pains, and can hurt the sinews. It should be avoided by old people, by people who are thin, and by melancholics.

Advice:
Vinegar made from good-quality wine is better than vinegar made from beer. In order to temper its negative qualities, roses, water or raisins can be added to it.

Since the medieval period, then, spices have been used across the globe – in medicine and in preparing meals – to rectify humoral imbalances in order to maintain or improve health. Proponents of the humoral system have stated categorically that using them has helped people of both genders and all ages, regardless of their lifestyles, to avoid or help cure specific health problems, and to aid natural bodily rhythms. But one needs to be careful about when and when not to use spices. While Robert Turner points out in *Botanologica the Brittish Physician* that substances like cinnamon are good for treating "cold and moist diseases," medical expert James Primerose in *Popular Errours* cautions against using spices if the patient has high fevers. This is because their natural heat exacerbates the problem. The inharmonious connection between eating spicy foods and fighting fevers was also commented on by head of state Oliver Cromwell in his advisory pamphlet addressed to carers of sick soldiers following the British Civil Wars. Primerose notes also that both diarrhea and excessive menstruation are ill-served by eating humorally hot and dry dishes made with spices. As Dr John Ball says in his 1770 medical guidebook entitled *The female physician: or, Every woman her own doctress*, menstrual blood is full of the choler humor; thus hot, dry substances might best be avoided by women at certain times during their monthly cycle.

Any disagreement between doctors revolved not around the

time-tested and approved theory of the humoral body, but rather which foods were best for maintaining and improving health – either locally produced plants or exotic ones. We have seen that while local herbs and vegetables have a broad range of humoral properties, spices and condiments are often "dry" and nearly always "hot." When made into sauces or added to meals, these substances typically act as an effective counterbalance to the opposite properties found in many types of flesh – such as young animals and birds and most species of fish. While poultry and fish are discussed in Chapter Seven, we look next at the benefits and dangers associated with eating animal flesh, dairy produce and eggs.

Chapter Six

Animal Flesh and Dairy Produce

A diet consisting of carefully selected fruits, vegetables and herbs is often sufficient to maintain one's health. But for those who prefer not to pursue a vegetarian or vegan lifestyle, we will now consider the humoral characteristics of a range of meats and dairy produce such as milk, cheese, cream, butter and eggs. Discussing the rights and wrongs of eating animal produce is beyond the scope of this book, and arguing the pros and cons of vegetarianism would in any case call for the publication of an inordinately large volume. Suffice it to say that highly trained doctors and expert nutritionists who brought to our table the concept of humorism and detailed descriptions of the health-fulness of foods were by no means insensitive to animal welfare. For example, Dr Thomas Moffett in his posthumous 1655 publi-cation *Healths Improvement* wrote that "all Birds feeding themselves abroad fat with wholesome meat, are of better nourishment than such as be cram'd in a coop or little house..." Vegetarianism also was a hot topic centuries ago, and works extolling the virtues of a meat-free diet range from *The English Hermite* by Roger Crab (published in the same year as Moffett's guidebook on healthy living) to *Emile* by the Geneva-born French philosopher Jean-Jacques Rousseau.

From a non-vegetarian's point of view, however, healthier animals, then as now, meant healthier food; and books on nutrition and healthful living written at that time show us that there are enough meats with different humoral characteristics to suit everyone – regardless of their constitution. Despite this, it needs to be borne in mind that many factors affect an animal's humoral characteristics, and that these are passed on to its consumer. For example, a free-range animal given good-quality, nutritious food will generate better meat than one confined to a small area and fed with poor-quality scraps. Furthermore, the meat of a young animal – say veal or young lamb – is humorally moister than beef or mutton. The younger the animal is, the more viscose its meat is likely to be as well. This is something that people with an overabundance of the phlegmatic humor need to watch out for. Eating this meat without "correcting" it can induce winter-related illnesses, and at the same time render one mentally less efficient. Similarly, a sheep or bull grazed on marshy land, or in a field next to a watercourse, is likely to be humorally cooler and moister than one dwelling on a mountainside. How do we know where the animal lived? Usually, unless we know the butcher, we don't. But another variable, one that is useful to us in this respect, is the length of time the carcass has been "aged." The longer it spends on the hook, the more its humoral balance shifts towards the center.

With all these variables at play, the characteristics described in this and the next chapter, and the advice given, can serve only as a brief but useful guide. I now call on the works of eminent scholars trained in medical humorism to show what the characteristics of animal meats and dairy products are understood to be.

Beef

Humoral property:
Cool in the first degree, dry in the second.

Positives:
This meat excels at nourishing the body. It generates good blood and prevents choleric humors from flowing around the body. Tender beef is particularly beneficial to young and active people in cold weather.

Negatives:
Beef is digested slowly, especially that which is sourced from bulls, and it therefore has the potential to be corrupted with ill humors when lying in the stomach. This can produce gastric problems in people who have relatively inactive lifestyles. Those with a melancholic temperament should avoid eating this meat without first correcting it with warming and drying additives such as mustard.

Advice:
The best beef is that which is tender and has been sourced from well-fed, two- to three-year-old animals. Young beef is best roasted; old beef is best boiled. Beef that has been salted is difficult to digest, and it engenders gross, melancholic humors that can be detrimental to health by lowering resistance to disease. Beef so treated should therefore be rinsed in water thoroughly before being cooked.

Chevon (goat flesh)

Humoral property:
Temperately warm, and moist in the first degree.

Positives:
The meat of young goats is easily and quickly digested, and it provides good nourishment. It is especially efficacious to people with weak constitutions, and those who are recovering from illness. It is also beneficial to young people and others with choleric humors.

Negatives:
The meat of old goats digests slowly and offers very little nourishment. Because of its humoral moistness, chevon should be avoided by the aged, and by people with cold stomachs or with an abundance of phlegmatic humors.

Advice:

The flesh of young red or black goats is thought to be the best. The hindquarters are more healthful than the forequarters on account of the latter's excessive humoral moistness. This meat is best eaten in the spring and early summer, and it is most nutritious after it has been roasted rather than boiled.

Hare

Humoral property:

Hot and dry in the second degree.

Positives:

Eaten in small quantities hare facilitates the production of a fit, slender body. It also produces a good fresh color in the face. Best eaten in winter, this meat is beneficial to youths and people with a sanguine constitution.

Negatives:

The meat of the hare is hard and humorally dry, it is not particularly nourishing, and it is digested slowly. It can engender melancholic humors. Eating too much of it at any one time may cause drowsiness. It is best avoided – especially by melancholics and people with an inactive lifestyle.

Advice:

Young, fat hares are more healthful than old, thin ones. Baste the meat with butter or lard, and bake rather than roast it.

Lamb

Humoral property:

Warm in the first degree, moist in the second. The flesh of young lambs is moist in the third degree.

Positives:

The meat of older lambs offers good and plentiful nourishment, and it helps to prevent the production of health-damaging melancholic humors. This meat is best for people with hot, dry constitutions such as youths and cholerics.

Negatives:

Young lamb is humorally moist to an excessive degree. Because of this it can cause stomach complaints and engender corrupt humors that leave the body susceptible to infection. It should thus be avoided – especially by old people and those who are phlegmatic.

Advice:

Male lambs, about a year old, are best. Their flesh should be roasted and eaten with hot herbs or spices such as rosemary, mint, garlic, sage or cloves.

Mutton

Humoral property:
Temperate in heat and moisture.

Positives:

This is an exceptionally good meat for nourishing the body. It is particularly efficacious to people with weak constitutions, and to convalescents. It can be eaten to promote good health at any time of the year, in any region, and by people of any age or constitution.

Negatives:

Mutton obtained from old sheep is slow in digestion and unwholesome. This is because it is overly dry and its humors have been corrupted with age.

Advice:
Choose the meat of young sheep that have been pastured on rich, fertile land. Ewe's meat is more nourishing than ram's meat. It is best boiled, not roasted, and eaten with herbs that open and clear blockages in the body.

Pork (farm-reared pigs)

Humoral property:
Warm in the first degree, moist in the second.

Positives:
Pork is a very nourishing meat, especially for people whose lifestyles require them to exercise and expend much energy. It keeps the digestive system in good working order, and it promotes the production and passing of urine in which gross, illness-inducing humors can be stored. It is an ideal food for consumption in cold weather, especially for young people and cholerics.

Negatives:
Because of its moistness and viscosity pork from young pigs can be detrimental to the health of inactive and old people, and to those with delicate stomachs. It is thought to engender gout and sciatica. It is best not to eat pork along with other meats at the same sitting, nor to eat the skin, which digests slowly.

Advice:
On account of their dubious humoral makeup, reject pork obtained from pigs that are either old or thin, and from pigs that have been factory farmed. Choose instead pork obtained from fully grown, free-range middle-aged male pigs, and roast rather than boil it. Meat from piglets contains much in the way of blockage-inducing phlegmatic humors and viscosity, and conse-quently it should be left alone or eaten in small quantities along

with spices or other humorally warm and moist foods.

Pork (wild boar)

Humoral property:
Warm and moist in the first degree.

Positives:
This meat is both very nourishing and easily digested. It is particularly suitable for people who are hot or who exercise greatly.

Negatives:
Like farm-produced pork, the meat of a wild boar is less beneficial to old people and others with an inactive lifestyle on account of its superfluous humors.

Advice:
Choose young and tender meat. It is most beneficial in cold weather, and should either be carved into steaks or baked as a joint with the addition of spices in order to reduce its humoral moistness.

Rabbit

Humoral property:
Slightly cool in the first degree, dry in the second.

Positives:
More humorally temperate than hare, rabbit offers very good nourishment. This meat aids the production and passing of urine, and removes excess phlegm and erodes corrupt humors that would otherwise attract any one of a variety of illnesses. It is most efficacious when eaten in warm weather, and is suitable for most people with sanguine, choleric or phlegmatic complexions.

Negatives:
On account of its dryness it might best be avoided by melancholics and old folk. This is particularly the case for older rabbits.

Advice:
Meat obtained from young, fat rabbits is the most beneficial to health – especially in the winter. Hang it for twenty-four hours in a cool place, then parboil it and roast it either with herbs or spice such as cloves.

Veal

Humoral property:
Temperate in all qualities.

Positives:
This meat is humorally well-balanced, it is easily and quickly digested which restricts the production of body-weakening gross humors, and it is very nourishing. It helps the body to produce good-quality blood, and it is particularly wholesome for people with active lifestyles. Veal is suitable to be eaten in all seasons of the year by people of all ages and most humoral constitutions.

Negatives:
The meat of very young animals is overly viscose. This may be harmful to phlegmatics, to people with weak constitutions, and to convalescents.

Advice:
Choose the meat of older animals that have been allowed to roam freely. Roast the meat rather than boil it, and add humorally warm and drying ingredients such as parsley.

Venison (fallow deer)

Humoral property:
Hot and dry in the second degree.

Positives:
This meat is more nourishing than venison obtained from other types of deer. It is beneficial to those who suffer from colic or palsy, and, unlike the meat from red deer, it can be eaten by melancholics. It is good for drying excess humors in phlegmatics.

Negatives:
This type of venison can dry the blood, and therefore should be avoided by thin people whose systems are easily harmed by hot, dry foods. The meat from old deer can irritate the sinews and the meat from fat deer can cause stomach upsets. Venison should be avoided by young people and others with an abundance of choler.

Advice:
Choose venison obtained from young deer that are neither too fat nor too thin. Make sure the meat is aged until it is tender, and then baste it thoroughly with oil or fat and roast it.

Venison (red deer)

Humoral property:
Warm in the first degree, dry in the second.

Positives:
Offering good nourishment, venison obtained from red deer is a healthful meat to those who possess cold- and moist-related characteristics, such as phlegmatics.

Negatives:

Venison is somewhat difficult to digest and can introduce corrupting humors to the body. This can leave one susceptible to infection. This meat is not recommended for consumption in hot weather – especially not for old people and melancholics.

Advice:

The meat from young red deer is best. Roast or bake it, and serve it with humorally warm, moist vegetables like asparagus or carrots.

In this chapter the discussion up until now has been about muscle flesh. But as offal is still popular in some quarters, I need to say a few words about the values and limitations of eating internal organs before I move on to dairy produce and eggs. Kidneys and liver are the most widely used organs in cooking these days, so I have concentrated only on these; but it may be noted that other internal organs of animals, and indeed of poultry, share similar humoral properties. Brain, for example, is exceedingly viscose and phlegmatic, and heart offers little nourishment and is difficult to digest.

Kidneys

Humoral property:

Cold in the second degree, moist in the third.

Positives:

This food is fit only for cholerics with strong stomachs. Kidneys of lambs, kids or piglets are the most nourishing.

Negatives:

Kidneys are even more difficult to digest than liver, they offer no good nourishment, and they contain gross humors. The older the animal is, the worse the humoral characteristics of the kidneys become. Phlegmatics should avoid this food.

Advice:
Choose the kidneys of a well-fed calf, or those of young smaller animals. Add spices or other drying ingredients.

Liver

Humoral property:
Cold and moist in the second degree.

Positives:
Liver can nourish those who are able to fully digest it. Livers taken from young poultry can clear the eyesight, increase blood production, and can be pleasing to the stomach.

Negatives:
This product is difficult to digest, and it engenders gross humors that can cause obstructions and leave the body susceptible to contracting illnesses. That which is obtained from animals – particularly old animals – is difficult to digest. Liver obtained from young animals is very phlegmatic.

Advice:
Choose livers from young animals and poultry, and correct them by cooking thoroughly with warm, dry ingredients.

Clearly, as far as maintaining good health is concerned – from a humoral angle at least – offal is probably best avoided by all but cholerics with "cast-iron" constitutions and outstanding digestive abilities. As we saw in Chapters Three to Five, vegetables and fruits – moderated where necessary with spices – provide all the nourishment we actually need; however, if one feels the need to eat animal meat, one is usually better off eating muscle meat. We now look at the nutritional values of a range of the more commonly eaten dairy products.

Butter

Humoral property:
Warm and moist in the first or second degree.

Positives:
Butter is good for removing phlegmatic humors from the breast and lungs. It cleans and strengthens the body and fights the symptoms of a cold – including relieving a cough. It is efficacious at any time of year, but no more so than in the morning; in the words of an old rhyme, butter is "gold in the morning, silver at noon, and lead in the evening." Because of its purging powers, butter is particularly beneficial to old people. It is also good for melancholics.

Negatives:
Eating too much butter weakens and loosens the stomach. This particularly is the case for people with sanguine characteristics.

Advice:
Sheep's butter is best. Choose fresh, sweet butter rather than old. In order to combat its viscose properties, butter should be eaten with strengthening and astringent foods.

Cheese (cottage or soft cheese)

Humoral property:
Cool and dry in the first degree.

Positives:
This dairy product is beneficial to people with hot constitutions, and cholerics suffering from slow or partial digestion. Soft cheese quenches the thirst, it fights choleric humors, and is beneficial to sanguines. It can be eaten at any time by people with a physically

active lifestyle.

Negatives:
Being slowly digested, it can irritate cold stomachs. It can make the eater feel sleepy.

Advice:
More nutritious than hard cheese, the best sort is that which is made with fresh, new milk.

Cheese (hard)

Humoral property:
Cold and moist in the second degree.

Positives:
Hard cheeses can reduce the level of excess humors in the body, and it is both nourishing and soothing. Eaten in moderation, it is very beneficial to youths, choleric people and those who have an active lifestyle.

Negatives:
Hard cheese binds the belly, and eating too much of it causes obstructions that can lock in putrefying humors. It is not suitable for phlegmatics and people with weak stomachs.

Advice:
Firm cheeses should be made from milk that humorally is as close to neutral as possible, and sourced from free-range cows, goats or sheep. Choose cheese that is young and fresh, for this has fewer corrupting humors. To rectify its few negative values, it may be eaten with nuts, pears or apples.

Cream

Humoral property:
Warm and moist in the first degree.

Positives:
Like butter, cream is excellent for cleansing the breast and preventing chest-related illnesses. It helps to neutralize gross humors in other foods, and it lines the stomach. It is most beneficial to young people, cholerics and others with hot stomachs.

Negatives:
Cream is only slowly absorbed by the body, and this can breed coarse, health-damaging humors when it is eaten after other foods. It should be avoided by old folk and people with rheumatism.

Advice:
Ideally, use freshly made cream wherever possible. Eat it sparingly with sour or humorally cool, moist food such as apples or strawberries, and temper these fruits further with either sugar, red wine or honey.

Eggs

Humoral property:
Temperate in heat and moisture.

Positives:
Humorally neutral, like the hen that laid them, eggs are the epitome of healthful food. They are rapidly digested and they greatly nourish the body. Eggs are beneficial to people with chest or stomach ailments, they open blockages in the digestive system enabling gross humors to be evacuated, and they can even clarify the voice. This food is also believed to have aphrodisiacal

powers. Good at all times of the year, eggs are suitable for all ages, constitutions and diseases.

Negatives:
Eggs can slow down the digestion of other foods if they are eaten straight after them. Eating too many eggs may cause skin blemishes.

Advice:
Freshly laid eggs of young hens are the most healthful. Although raw eggs are more quickly digested, and therefore less likely to cause health problems, boiled or poached eggs are the more nutritious – especially the yolks (the whites are humorally cooler and moister). Hard, fried eggs are less nourishing and can produce gross humors that can corrupt other foods lying in the stomach. Eggs are best eaten on their own.

Milk

Humoral property:
Moist in the second degree, temperate in heat.

Positives:
Milk enhances the mental faculties, and it admirably nourishes the body. It is also good for the production and passing of urine, and it is a mild aphrodisiac. Closest to the humoral properties of blood itself, milk is an ideal food during hot weather, and is particularly beneficial to children, old people, cholerics and others with hot stomachs.

Negatives:
People should avoid milk if they are suffering from an infection of the blood, a headache, or sore eyes. It should also be omitted from the diet of people who have kidney complaints, obstructions in the digestive system, or toothache.

Advice:

The milk of grazing animals living on rich pastures away from marshes and fens is the best – especially in the spring and early summer. Choose cow's milk first, sheep's second and goat's milk third. To get the maximum benefit out of milk, either use it for cooking or, if it is for drinking, add a little honey, salt, sugar or mint to prevent it from curdling in the stomach and producing crude humors. It is best to drink it on an empty stomach in order to prevent the body from producing melancholic humors.

As is the case for vegetables and herbs, there are enough types of animal produce to cater for everyone's dietary needs. This is because they possess between them a range of humoral attributes that cover the entire spectrum of healthful eating. But eating a type of meat that at face value appears to be incongruous with one's humoral makeup need not be a problem. It depends on how it is cooked and what is eaten with it. Examples of humoral rectification dating back centuries are still with us to this day: warm, moist lamb is sometimes served with mint sauce – the vinegar being cooling and drying; roast beef that is humorally cold is warmed with mustard; and warm, moist pork may be "corrected" with apple sauce made from cool, dry cooking apples such as Bramleys.

Four-legged animals and dairy produce, however, are not the only source of nourishment available to non-vegetarians and non-vegans. There is also poultry and fish to consider, and the humoral characteristics and medical nutritional values of these foods are discussed in the next chapter.

Chapter Seven

Birds and Aquatic Foods

For those who eat meat, the value of poultry in restoring good health has been widely recognized for a long time. Lighter, finer in texture, and more easily digested than "red" meats, poultry is often fed to those who are convalescing. Even centuries ago doctors advised patients suffering from a whole range of illnesses to eat chicken broth. A few of the many examples can be found in *An Alphabetical Book of Physicall Secrets* written by professor of medicine Owen Wood and published in 1639. It is not just the lightness and digestibility of birds that favorably impressed these medical experts; for they understood also that restoring humoral balance is pivotal to recovery, and that chicken flesh – like the hen's egg – is the epitome of humoral moderation. Not all birds share the same medical characteristics, however; and no matter what the patient's humoral constitution might be, there is light, easily digested bird meat that can be prepared in some way or another to maintain or improve a person's health.

Fish and other aquatic lifeforms are different. Books written by experts in humoral medicine show that, as far as health is concerned, this source of nourishment is often damagingly viscose and sometimes on the "cold" and "moist" side of the "golden mean" – even after having been cooked. They inform their readers that freshwater fish in general, and pond-dwelling fish in particular, are not really good for people who feel unwell. They also say that saltwater fish, if eaten at all, has to be eaten in moderation. Despite this the learned authors go to great lengths to point out that fishes, like birds, possess a range of character-istics – any of which might be more suited to the dietary needs of one person than to another. This chapter considers the attributes of these types of food as seen from the humoral angle.

Chicken

Humoral property:
Temperate in heat and moisture.

Positives:
Chicken nourishes the body more than any other meat. It generates good temperate humors and is good for the chest, stomach and brain. It is suitable for any age and constitution, particularly for people who get limited amounts of physical exercise. It can usefully be eaten at any time, and its recuperative powers for those who are ill are excellent – especially in the summer. Medicinally it is good for treating gout, aching joints and fevers.

Negatives:
People with cool, moist constitutions should note that young pullets have phlegmatic qualities, and cholerics should be aware that cockerels are humorally hotter than hens.

Advice:
Young, well-fed birds are the most efficacious. Eat chicken moderately, and combine this with taking exercise.

Duck

Humoral property:
Hot and moist in the second degree.

Positives:
Duck is very nourishing, particularly the flesh from fat birds. It is good for the complexion, it clears the throat, it increases male fertility, and it disperses wind that would otherwise corrupt the humors and attract illness. This bird is best eaten in cold weather,

and is beneficial to melancholics.

Negatives:
It is difficult to digest, it can introduce phlegmatic humors to the body, and it offers little nourishment to hot people. Older ducks can induce fever in cholerics.

Advice:
The most healthful ducks are young and tender but well fed. The foreparts are the most nourishing. The duck's heat may be moderated by eating it with cooling herbs such as borage.

Goose

Humoral property:
Warm in the first degree, moist in the second.

Positives:
The flesh of a gosling is somewhat nourishing and helps to stem weight loss. Like duck, it is best eaten in cold weather by people with physically active lifestyles.

Negatives:
The meat of this bird is digested slowly and fills the body with superfluous humors. Older geese are humorally hotter than goslings, and this may attract fevers in choleric people.

Advice:
Free-range geese that are young and well fed are beneficial to health. The meat of this bird is best roasted with cooling herbs.

Partridge

Humoral property:
Warm in the first degree, dry in the second.

Positives:

This bird is easily digested, which prevents the corruption of humors that have the potential to cause illness. It also provides excellent nourishment and actually dries superfluous humors in the stomach. Furthermore, partridge is thought to sharpen the mental faculties, to increase fertility, and to act as a mild aphrodisiac. Partridge is a particularly useful addition to the diet of people recovering from illness, and can be eaten by all but cholerics – especially in cold weather.

Negatives:

It can cause choler-related problems in people with humorally hot constitutions. Old birds are tougher, hotter and less easy to digest.

Advice:

Young, female partridges are thought to be the best. Older birds should be hung up for twenty-four hours to moderate their humoral heat.

Pheasant

Humoral property:
Temperate in heat and moisture.

Positives:

Very nourishing, pheasant is good for the stomach, reduces the effects of fever, and strengthens convalescents. Best eaten in the autumn, this bird is suitable for people of all humoral constitutions.

Negatives:

Eating too much of it can make one short-winded.

Advice:
Fat pheasants are the best, but they are humorally dryer than chicken and best eaten with moistening foods.

Pigeon

Humoral property:
Hot and moist in the second degree.

Positives:
The meat of this bird is readily digested. It can help to relieve the symptoms of palsy in humorally cold people such as melancholics, and it usefully increases the heat in them. It purges the kidneys of gross humors, and it is thought to have aphrodisiacal powers. Best eaten in cold weather, pigeon meat is particularly beneficial to the health of melancholics, old people and phlegmatics.

Negatives:
Pigeons can inflame the blood and can adversely affect the heads and stomachs of cholerics and other hot people.

Advice:
Fat pigeons are the best. In order to moderate their humors they should be boiled in the gravy of other meats and eaten with drying ingredients like verjuice, vinegar and coriander, and cooling ingredients like plums or cherries.

Quail

Humoral property:
Hot in the first or second degree, moist in the second degree.

Positives:
This bird is most useful to melancholics because it neutralizes their humoral dryness. It is beneficial to them when it is eaten in

cold weather.

Negatives:
Digested slowly, quail readily corrupts the humors in the stomach. This can cause aches and cramps, and can leave the body susceptible to contracting fevers. It may be most harmful to the aged and to phlegmatics.

Advice:
Young, tender and fat ones are the best. They should be eaten with drying foods like coriander or vinegar to mollify their humoral moisture.

Turkey

Humoral property:
Hot and moist in the second degree.

Positives:
Turkey offers plenty of good nourishment. Despite its heat and moisture it tends to correct humoral balance and strengthen the body. It is an excellent restorative food for people who are recovering from illness. It is thought to increase fertility and at once act as a mild aphrodisiac. This bird is beneficial to health at any time of the year, and it is suitable for all people except the very old and infirm.

Negatives:
Eating too much turkey can leave inactive people with gout, and it can cause defluxions. The meat of this bird can be overly fattening compared to chicken.

Advice:
Young, well-fed free-range turkeys are the most efficacious. To moderate their humoral properties they should be hung up to

age, and then roasted with drying spices. Eat this meat only occasionally, and a little at a time. The breast is the most nutritious part.

We now turn our attention to the medical properties of some of the more commonly eaten aquatic life – including saltwater and freshwater fish, molluscs and crustaceans. Fish has held a significant place in sustaining humans since the earliest of times. It is mentioned as an allowable and useful source of nourishment to humans in major holy texts such as the Quran and the Christian Bible, and its value as a source of nourishment is acknowledged by modern nutritionists, by doctors of old, and by ancient medical writers. The nutritional value of fish when eaten as a staple, and its economic importance, are still widely appreciated in coastal communities, and it can be found posturing as a luxury in high-end restaurants. If we eat it, then, what could possibly go wrong? The answer to that depends on the consumer's own particular humoral composition, lifestyle and age, and the characteristics of the fish being eaten. Thus, this source of food can be medicinal or it can bring to the surface any underlying health problem. This is what guidebooks written by the foremost proponents of humoral medicine have to say about obtaining, preparing and eating various aquatic foods:

Carp

Humoral property:
Of temperate heat, moist in the first degree.

Positives:
Carp is more nourishing than other freshwater fish. Those living in rivers are more wholesome than those living in ponds. This fish can safely be eaten by people of any age or humoral complexion at any time of year.

Negatives:
The beneficial qualities of carp tend to deteriorate if the fish is kept for a long time before eating it.

Advice:
Fry it in oil and serve it with drying herbs, vinegar or spices.

Cockles and Mussels

Humoral property:
Warm in the first degree, moist in the second.

Positives:
They stimulate the appetite, and, despite their mild heat, they can be eaten by cholerics.

Negatives:
Both of these molluscs, and especially mussels, are inferior to oysters insofar as they offer very little nourishment and are relatively difficult and slow to digest. They can cause obstructions in the body that can putrefy humors and engender illnesses.

Advice:
Select cockles and/or mussels that come from clear rather than murky waters. Eat them only occasionally between autumn and spring, and in very modest quantities. Prepare them with pepper and vinegar to dry their humors.

Cod

Humoral property:
Cool and moist in the first degree.

Positives:
Fresh cod is of moderate firmness and is nourishing. It is beneficial to youths, to people with hot constitutions, and to

cholerics.

Negatives:
Glutinous, clammy and cold, this fish is not easily digested. It can induce phlegmatic humors in the body, and is best avoided by people with cold constitutions – especially in the winter. Salted cod dries the humors but makes the fish even harder to digest.

Advice:
Choose medium-sized fish, and cook and eat it in moderation with humorally drying ingredients such as oil, vinegar, salt or parsley.

Crab

Humoral property:
Cold in the second degree, moist in the first.

Positives:
Eating the meat from a crab can help to fight chest complaints, and it can help to prevent the spread of infections arising from insect or animal bites. Eating crab stimulates the passing of urine and cleans the kidneys, and this meat is also said to have aphrodisiacal powers. This is a good food for cholerics.

Negatives:
Although it is nourishing, it is digested only slowly. It engenders gross phlegmatic humors and should be avoided by people with cold constitutions.

Advice:
Crabs harvested from freshwater sources are more nutritious than sea crabs. They are best in early spring and late summer, especially when caught and eaten when the moon is full. Roast a

crab quickly and eat it with vinegar and pepper that corrects its humoral moistness.

Crayfish

As for **Crab**.

Eel

Humoral property:
Slightly cool in the first degree, moist in the first degree.

Positives:
Eel is very nourishing. It has a long shelf life when it is salted, and eating this food helps to stem the buildup of phlegmatic humors in the stomach. When eaten in moderate quantities, eel can be beneficial to people of all ages and constitutions.

Negatives:
Fat eels in particular have clammy, glutinous humors that can cause obstructions and engender gout and stones. Eel is also a little windy. The back of an eel is less beneficial to health than the front of it.

Advice:
Choose eels that have been caught in the sea, not in a muddy estuary or a fen. The latter have gross humors. They are best cooked and eaten in the spring, immediately after having been caught. To moderate its humors roast the eel in paper, with oil and warm, drying herbs like sage, parsley or coriander; alternatively keep it salted for a day or two and add some oregano. Eat it sparingly, and with vinegar.

Flat fish (flounder, plaice, sole, turbot)

Humoral property:
Cool and moist in the first degree. Young plaice and flounders are

moist in the second degree.

Positives:
This type of fish is easily digested and offers good nourishment, especially sole which is excellent for both healthy and sick people. The turbot's firmness makes it a good food for people with an active lifestyle.

Negatives:
Although plaice and flounder are generally wholesome, small, young specimens are watery and full of phlegmatic humors which, on account of their illness-inducing properties, make them unsuitable for old people and those with weak stomachs.

Advice:
Choose firm ones, but reject those that are old. Cook them in oil with drying foods while they are still fresh, and eat them with drying herbs.

Haddock
Similar properties to cod (above), except that it is softer and more easily digested.

Halibut
Humoral property:
Warm in the first degree, moist in the second.

Positives:
Firm and white, this fish is nutritious. It is particularly suitable for people who have strong stomachs, it cools the blood, and it can be eaten by cholerics and others with hot constitutions.

Negatives:
It is slowly digested and has glutinous, moist humors that can

harm the stomachs of phlegmatics.

Advice:
Young halibut is best. Eat small quantities only in the summer, and avoid eating freshly caught halibut in the winter due to its phlegmatic qualities. To mollify its humoral moistness boil it gently in water and vinegar, and eat it with vinegar and drying herbs.

Herring

Humoral property:
Cool and moist in the first degree.

Positives:
This fish is easily digested, and when eaten in moderation it is nutritious. Suitable for physically active people and cholerics, it may also be eaten in small quantities by people with weak stomachs.

Negatives:
Fresh, very young herrings are overly moist; salted or pickled herrings are dryer and more difficult to digest.

Advice:
Choose the fat ones that have firm flesh. Cook them with a sprinkling of salt, or in water and vinegar, to correct their humors.

Lamprey

Humoral property:
Temperate heat, moist in the first degree.

Positives:
Its near-temperate qualities make the lamprey nutritious. It is digested rapidly which helps to inhibit the production of putre-

fying humors, and it is believed to aid fertility in men. It can safely be eaten at any time of year, and is beneficial to the health of all but old and infirm people.

Negatives:
Undercooked lamprey is digested only slowly, and this engenders gross humors that cause illness. It should not be eaten by people with gout or inflamed sinews.

Advice:
River lamprey is best. It should be eaten in March or April. Cook it in humorally drying white wine, oil and spices.

Lobster

Humoral property:
Cool and moist in the first degree.

Positives:
Lobster exhibits similar properties to crab (above), but lobster is less cold. This makes eating it more appropriate to people with phlegmatic humors.

Negatives:
This marine crustacean is difficult to digest, and therefore the humors lying in the stomach can putrefy. These corrupt humors may then engender stomach upsets.

Advice:
As for **Crab** (above).

Mackerel

Humoral property:
Cool in the first degree, moist in the second or third.

Positives:
Having reasonably firm flesh, mackerel is sweet and nutritious to all but those who have an overabundance of phlegmatic humors. It is particularly beneficial to people with hot constitutions and to those who have a physically active lifestyle.

Negatives:
Its viscosity and moistness engenders gross humors in the stomachs of those with sedentary lifestyles. Mackerel should be avoided by sick people.

Advice:
Eat young, fresh mackerel that are not too small. Prepare the fish by cooking it with humorally drying ingredients.

Mullet

Humoral property:
Warm in the first degree, dry in the second.

Positives:
Mullet is best used externally. Applied to a flesh wound, it helps to cure infections and resists poison. It is best eaten in hot weather by youths, cholerics and others with humorally hot stomachs.

Negatives:
This fish is difficult to digest, and lingers long in the stomach. This can cause abdominal ailments. Drinking the wine in which mullet has been cooked suppresses sex drive and reduces fertility both in men and women.

Advice:
The smaller fish caught in clear, moving water are better than the ones taken from standing or muddy waters. To moderate their

humoral properties either sprinkle them with oil or orange juice and roast them, or boil them in vinegar with sweet herbs.

Oyster

Humoral property:
Warm in the first degree, moist in the second.

Positives:
Oysters may be eaten by young people with strong stomachs and by those with an abundance of choler – but only from autumn to spring. Easy to digest, this shellfish loosens the belly if eaten before meals, stimulates the appetite, and has mild aphrodisiacal powers.

Negatives:
Despite being humorally moist its juice has a high salt content. Oysters are not particularly nourishing. They greatly increase phlegm in cold stomachs and cause obstructions which can generate sickness.

Advice:
Eat very few oysters, and choose only those that have been harvested from clear waters. Reject oysters that have been taken from muddy waters. Preparing these molluscs with pepper and the juice of sour oranges or vinegar dries and cools their humors.

Pike

Humoral property:
Cold and moist in the second degree.

Positives:
The meat of the pike is hard, and therefore it is best eaten in the winter. Due to its humoral qualities pike is beneficial only to people with strong digestive systems and choleric constitutions.

Negatives:
Pike offers little nourishment, it is difficult for the body to digest, and it lies long in the stomach. Along with its phlegmatic qualities this can leave the body susceptible to contracting illnesses, and its humoral dampness may also adversely affect the mental faculties. It should be eaten neither by those who are sick nor by people who have sedentary lifestyles.

Advice:
Avoid eating pike that have been taken from ponds. Large, fat pike caught in clear rivers are best. Pike should be cooked and eaten straight away. To mollify its corrupting humors it should be boiled gently with sweet herbs and oil, and eaten with white vinegar and marjoram.

Pilchards

Humoral property:
Cool in the first degree, moist in the first or second degree.

Positives:
Fresh pilchards are quickly digested, so there is little time for them to adversely affect other foods lying in the stomach. This fish also offers some nourishment.

Negatives:
Similar to herrings; but pilchards are sweeter and more viscose and moist. Therefore, if they are eaten in immoderate quantities they engender gross humors that can attract illnesses. Salted and pickled pilchards contain more bad humors, and they are more difficult to digest and less nourishing. These should be avoided by cholerics and melancholics.

Advice:
Drink humorally warm, moist beverages like red wine while

eating them.

Prawns and Shrimps

Humoral property:
Cool and moist in the first degree.

Positives:
These crustaceans provide good, wholesome nourishment – more so than the molluscs discussed above like cockles, oysters and mussels. They are quickly and easily digested which helps to prevent a buildup of excess humors. They are suitable for any age and humoral constitution, and can be particularly beneficial to young, active people, and to those who have choleric temperaments.

Negatives:
Eating too many can cause obstructions in the digestive system and attract gross humors that can bring about illness.

Advice:
Avoid eating prawns or shrimps that have been taken from muddy or polluted waters. Those harvested from clear water are best. Prepare them in oil or vinegar to aid humoral balance.

Sturgeon

Humoral property:
Warm in the first degree, moist in the second.

Positives:
This is a reasonably nourishing fish. Despite being warm in the first degree, sturgeon can help to cool the humors in the blood, and eating a small quantity of this fish is thought to increase one's sex drive. It may be eaten by all except those with hot stomachs and inflamed joints, and it is particularly beneficial to

melancholics.

Negatives:
As it is slowly digested, it can produce gross, cloying humors. This particularly is the case for fat sturgeon. The flesh of this fish in general, and that taken from the back of the fish in particular, should not be eaten by sick people, by those who are convalescing, or by melancholics.

Advice:
Young sturgeon sourced from rivers rather than from the sea are best. Eat the belly of this fish in the summer, and in small quantities only. To correct its humoral properties boil it gently in water and vinegar, and eat it with white vinegar and cinnamon or fennel.

Tench

Humoral property:
Cold and moist in the second degree.

Positives:
Tench offers little in the way of nourishment, but medically, if it is cut lengthways and applied to the soles of the feet, it can help to relieve a fever. It may be eaten by youths, cholerics and hot people with active lifestyles, but ideally only in the autumn or winter.

Negatives:
It is slowly digested and lingers long in the stomach. This engenders illness-inducing cold, gross humors. It should not be eaten in the summer, and never by phlegmatics.

Advice:
Avoid eating tench that has been sourced from ponds, and eat

only those caught in rivers. Dry bake it with humorally drying ingredients such as garlic, sweet herbs and spices; or, if it is to be boiled, boil it with oil, onion and humorally warming spices or raisins.

Trout

Humoral property:
Slightly cool in the first degree, moist in the first or second degree.

Positives:
This fish is easily digested and it is very nutritious. Its moderate coolness rectifies an overly hot liver, and eating it cleanses the blood. It is beneficial to people with fevers, and it can be eaten in hot weather by people of all ages and humoral complexions except the very old, infirm and phlegmatics.

Negatives:
Trout flesh can corrupt the humors of people with weak stomachs.

Advice:
This fish is best caught and eaten while it is still fresh between late April and early June. Eat only plump trout caught in fast-flowing streams, and never those taken from pools. Gently boil the fish in water and drying vinegar, and eat it with a sour sauce.

While the heat of poultry usually ranges from temperate to warm, and the flesh of birds generally is valued for its health-restoring properties, many fish are cold, moist and viscose. This means that some aquatic lifeforms can generate health-damaging phlegmatic humors, especially when they are eaten in cool, damp conditions. As is the case for animal flesh, however, the characteristics of fish can be "corrected." The botanist and physician Nicholas Culpeper observed that in his day "people usually boyl Fennel with Fish, and know not why they do it but only for custom." He explained that the origin of that practice "was founded upon Reason, because Fennel consumes that Flegmatick quality of Fish, which is obnoxious to the Body of man." Even to this day, without realizing the medical reasoning that lies behind our customary practices, many of us "correct" the humors of our fish before eating it. A sprinkle of vinegar and a slice of lemon have in the past acted, and still do act, as "drying" agents to a clammy or oily piece of fish. Parsley sauce goes one better; it is hot and dry, and therefore neutralizes the fish's coldness as well.

As is the case for the other foods discussed in this book, there are far too many types of birds and fish to include them all. I do believe, however, that by referring to the descriptions of the foods that feature throughout these pages, it is possible to make an informed choice about which ones to eat in order to maintain and improve one's health. All of the items discussed so far – meats, vegetables, fruits, spices etc. – are not just here for our sustenance or enjoyment; they are far more than that. Every mouthful of every meal does something to our bodies. Depending on each food's characteristics, it acts with or reacts against another to shore up, fine-tune or subtly change our constitution. Thus, every single food item discussed in this and the previous chapters is actually a *medicine*. There are times, however, when a small concentrated dose of a substance (usually made from herbs or fruits) is needed to rapidly put right something that has gone wrong. How to make these substances, and what to do with them, is discussed next.

Part III – Short Term Cures

Chapter Eight

Make Your Own Medicines

Food *is* medicine. As we have seen, regulating one's health is largely a matter of eating balanced meals that have been cleverly planned. The foods that go into dishes; how they are cooked; the ingredients that are added to them; the order in which they are eaten; the time of day; the time of year... These are main considerations in our quest to stay healthy or purge our bodies of illness-generating superfluous or tainted humors. But sometimes we need to go beyond this. We occasionally need to take more drastic action to rid our bodies of maladies that stubborn, corrupted humors have attracted. This involves taking small doses of medicine to eradicate infection, to cleanse the system, and ultimately to re-establish humoral balance. Making medicines to do this is not as difficult as one might think.

In the days before chemical and mineral compounds were introduced, and before the medical profession was mystified – be it to establish and secure the prestige of practitioners, or to justify the high price of drugs, or for any other reason – medicines were often made at home. Thankfully, doctors in those days were open about how to make them (more so than pharmacists who had a vested interest in selling lotions and potions), and wrote books telling people in plain, simple language how to do it.

Based squarely on the humoral system, the ingredients they say should be used are commonly found in household kitchens, gardens, or in the countryside. Mainly they are the herbs, fruits and spices discussed in Chapters Three to Five of this book. The medical recipes that follow come both from these publications and from diaries and handwritten notebooks (known as commonplace books) kept by women who were in charge of their families' health. But do these medicines actually work?

Thankfully I have not had occasion to try most of them – apart from the recipes for treating a cold (method 2), a chesty cough and a new cough, which, like eating a portion of pineapple, seems to work admirably for me – and so I cannot verify or dispute the effectiveness of the others. But comments accompanying notebook recipes testify that the medicines to which they refer were actually made, tried and tested, and are indeed fit for purpose. Typical observations include those made by English housekeepers Elizabeth Shirley of Radgate in Leicestershire and Elizabeth Barkham of Maxstoke in Warwickshire. While Shirley insists her medicine for curing fevers "hardly ever fails," and her water for expelling kidney stones is "marvellous good," Barkham describes her cure for melancholy as "an excellent syrup." Those who had their medical works published also were enthusiastic about the effectiveness of their medicines. In *An hospitall for the diseased*, for example, the author T. C. (possibly Thomas Cartwright) said in 1579 that his recipe for "the extreme cough" is "An excellent medicine."

As I stressed earlier in this book, individuals have different humoral characteristics and bodily requirements; so what works perfectly well for one person may not be efficacious to another. We see this today in the effectiveness (or lack of effectiveness) of different brands of commercially available cough medicine, for example. Doctors well versed in humoral medicine were well aware of individuality, and it is not uncommon to find several alternative recipes in one medical guidebook for treating the same illness.

Here are the details of making and taking medicines, as recommended by these medical experts of former times, and by "end users" (patients and their carers). Because there is a possibility that following the guidelines described below – or following guidelines expressed anywhere else for that matter – may not be in the best interest of the patient, one should seek professional advice before administering any medicines, or use one's own judgment, and improvise where necessary. In the best tradition of humoral medicine, one should also take into account the patient's personal complexion and dietary requirements.

Symptoms and common names of illnesses are listed in alphabetical order below, and the expressions contained within quotation marks (" ") are those of the original authors.

Aches and strains

Mix together one ounce each of marjoram and pennyroyal, and a handful each of bay leaves, chamomile flowers and lavender. Add to this a large nutmeg and some mace (a derivative of nutmeg), and the rind of four lemons and four oranges. Pulp all these ingredients together until it is a fine texture, and add a quarter of a pint of Malaga (fortified wine) and half a pound of unsalted butter. Bottle it and take as necessary.

Ague

See **Fever**.

Apoplexy

Drink every morning half a pint of distilled lavender water, and rub the head vigorously every morning and evening with a very clean, coarse cloth. By doing this the humors are dissolved and dispersed to the outward parts of the body. Furthermore, you should keep your feet and the nape of your neck warm and dry to prevent pain from recurring. Inhaling the strong scent of a fox is thought by some to be effective.

Appetite, loss of

To restore lost appetite take a handful of each of these: wormwood, mint, sage, cumin powder and brown bread. Pound it all together, put it in a linen cloth, and dampen it with vinegar. Heat it up as hot as you can stand and place it on your stomach.

Asthma

Make a stock medicine by crushing a pound of garlic into a fine pulp, adding to it the juice of six oranges and six lemons, straining it off, and mixing it with a general tonic. Take one spoonful of the liquid night and morning.

Backache

Clean and crush some burr roots, and put them in stale ale. Boil it well and strain it, discarding the sediment. Drink it cold in the morning and hot at night.

Baldness

Take hazelnuts, with husks and all, and burn them until they turn to powder. Then take beech mast and the leaves of elecampane (horse-heal flower), and crush the whole lot together. Gently boil it all with honey, and apply it to the bald area. Also, sprinkle some of the powder on the area. "This will make hair grow."

Bite, animal (1)

Crush walnuts, salt and an onion in a mortar. Apply the paste to the animal bite.

Bite, animal (2)

Lay some fresh, green betony (a grassland herb) on the bite. This may help "in very short space."

Bite, animal (3)

Mix urine-producing herbs such as violets, parsley and fennel that help to expel poison with either oxymel (diluted honey) or lemon syrup.

Bite, mosquito

Smear lemon juice onto exposed areas of the skin to deter insects from biting.

Bite, venomous creatures (1)

Crush some garlic and apply it to the bite, "and it will in short time cure the same." Also, eating garlic may cleanse the body and purify the blood.

Bite, venomous creatures (2)

Mix the powder of *Aristolochia rotunda* (smearwort) with the juice of mint, and apply it to the wound.

Bite, venomous creatures (3)

Crush the root of bruisewort (comfrey) and apply it to the wound to "heal the biting of venomous beasts."

Breastfeeding, insufficient milk (1)

To increase a woman's milk, boil some colewort in strong posset-ale (hot milk that has been curdled in ale), and drink some of it at every mealtime. Eat some colewort with each meal.

Breastfeeding, insufficient milk (2)

Drink the juice of vervain or fennel oftentimes, "and she shall have great plenty of milk."

Breath, bad (1)

If one suffers from bad breath one should make a medicine by distilling oak buds, and drink the juice every morning and evening for nine days. After a break, it should be taken again.

Breath, bad (2)

To rid the mouth of evil breath one should chew and suck cloves.

Breath, shortness of

Take two ounces of almond oil (extracted by crushing the nuts);

one ounce of fresh, unsalted butter; a little saffron; and fresh beeswax. Make an ointment by mixing these together. Apply this to the chest evening and morning.

Breathing difficulty, due to overweight
To help an overweight person breathe more easily, toast unleavened bread, dip it in clarified honey, and feed it to the patient several times along with his or her meals.

Burns or scalds (1)
Put the white of an egg in a pewter dish, and beat it until it is frothy. Then take fine cloth, dampen it in olive or vegetable oil, and place the cloth on the burned or scalded skin. Place the egg white on top of the cloth to draw out the heat and heal the sore.

Burns or scalds (2)
Take the yolks from four hardboiled eggs and gently fry them in a pan until they turn black. Take the oil that comes out of these black yolks and seal it in a container. This should be applied to the affected area as and when required.

Burns or scalds (3)
Whisk olive oil and a little water until the liquor turns white. Apply this to the sore area.

Cataracts
Take a good handful of marigold plants, a handful of fennel, and a handful of mayweed (chamomile). Crush them together, strain them with a pint of beer, and put it into a sealed container. Let the patient drink this when he or she is in bed, lying on the side where the cataract is, and drink it again in the morning.

Chest pains, relief for
Pound a good quantity of ripe sloes in a mortar, and put the fruit

in an earthenware container full of new ale. Drink this as and when it is required.

Cold (1)

Take seeds of the nettle plant, and simmer them in oil. Apply the lotion to the feet and hands.

Cold (2)

Mix together licorice, sugar, aniseeds, white wine vinegar, and lemon juice. Take a little as necessary.

Cold and cough

Take hyssop (a herb with antiseptic properties), rosemary, plantain and radish roots, and boil them gently in four pints of wine. When it has reduced to two pints, take out the herbs, pound the juice out of them, and strain the juice back into the wine. Then boil a pint of honey, remove the scum, add to it a quarter of a pound of clarified butter, and simmer for two minutes. Strain the whole through a linen cloth and put the liquor in a sealed container. The patient should take this first thing in the morning and last thing at night with six spoonfuls of warm, stale ale, until he or she is better – "for this is a proved medicine."

Colic

Distill some parsley water, add it to white wine or good ale, and drink it.

Cough, chesty

Take four pints of water, twenty figs, four ounces of refined sugar, a "good" quantity of licorice and aniseed, a small quantity of maidenhair (fern), and a handful of raisins. Boil them until two pints are left (reduce by half) and seal the liquor in a container. A little of it should be heated up and given to the patient to drink as required.

Cough, children's

Mix together half an ounce of sweet almond oil, half an ounce of diacodium (poppy syrup) and the juice of a lemon. Thicken the mixture with double-refined sugar.

Cough, extreme

Take washed fennel roots, some aniseeds and a little licorice, and boil them gently in white wine. Drink a good draft of this at bedtime and in the next morning. It is helpful also to roast a fig and a date, and eat them hot; but neither eat nor drink for two or three hours after.

Cough, mild

Take sage, rue (herb of grace) and pepper, and gently boil them with honey. Eat a spoonful both first thing in the morning and last thing at night until the cough has gone.

Cough, new

Take a spoonful of sugar and add to it, a drop at a time, the best aqua vitae (spirit such as brandy, whisky etc.) until the sugar is saturated. Then, when it is time to go to bed, eat the spoonful of sugar and cover yourself with warm bedding. This will "soon break and dissolve the cold."

Cough, old

If the cough is stubborn and lingering, seemingly fixed to the lungs, follow this procedure: Take two drams each of finely powdered betony, caraway seeds, pepper and hounds tongue (of the borage family). Mix them together with clarified honey and drink it morning and evening for nine days.

You may also take beaten candied sugar, an ounce each of finely chopped licorice, aniseeds and coriander seeds, mix them together and keep them in a bag in your pocket. When necessary you may eat a pinch of this to ease your cough.

Cramp (1)

Mix oil of chamomile with fenugreek, and apply it to the place where the cramp is.

Cramp (2)

Mix together and boil some betony, wormwood, vervain, and thyme. Put the liquid in a bath and lie in it, making sure to wash the area where the cramp is.

Dandruff (1)

Wash your hair often with either the essence of mallow roots (extracted by boiling them) or with the essence of the inner bark of elm.

Dandruff (2)

Wash the hair, and then apply vinegar and wine boiled together.

Dizziness, or swimming head

Mix together two drams each of agnus castus, broomwort, dried chamomile, oil of roses and white wine until it is thick. Stick this substance to the temples of the head "and it will in short space take away the grief."

Drunkenness, prevention of

Take powder of betony and colewort and mix them together. Eat one level teaspoon of it every morning before breakfast, "and it will preserve a man from drunkenness."

Earache (1)

Mix together the juices extracted from betony with oil of roses. Warm it up and place a few drops in the ears.

Earache (2)

Mix together oil of roses and a little vinegar, and apply it to the ears. Then place a cloth bag containing chamomile and melilot on the ears.

Ear infection

Take two handfuls of sage, one handful of hyssop (a herb with antiseptic properties) and half a handful of rosemary. Boil them in rose vinegar, rosewater and aqua vitae and put them in a cloth bag. Heat the bag as hot as you can stand, and place it on the ear.

Eyes, dimness of sight

Extract the juice from one of the following: hounds tongue (of the borage family), centaury (an antioxidant plant), sanicle, or sunflower, and apply it to the eyes "that be almost blynde and it shall help them."

Eyes, discharge

Mix together dried, powdered sage, powdered sea salt, and finely grated nutmeg. Place them in a linen bag, heat it up, and hold it on the nape of the neck.

Eyes, sore

For sore or bloodshot eyes, beat the white of an egg, and mix it with the same quantity of rosewater and the same quantity of juice of houseleek (*Sempervivum*). Then dip flat "pleageants" into the mix and place them on the sore eyes. Repeat as necessary until the eyes are better.

Fever (1)

Take a handful of bay leaves, a handful or more of red sage (Chinese sage), and gently boil them in four pints of stale ale until the liquor is reduced by half. Strain it, discarding the sodden herbs, warm it, add a little sugar, and drink "a good draught" while in bed.

Fever (2)

Put a handful each of parsley, fennel, centaury and pimpernel in four pints of weak ale. Boil it until it is reduced by half. Drink some of it as and when required.

Fever (3)

Extract the juice of an equal quantity of endives, sow thistle (*Sonchus*), dandelion, lettuce and sorrel, and distill them all together.

Fever, intermittent

Put a large spoonful of salt of wormwood (carbonate of potash) in a basin, and squeeze upon it the juice of a large lemon. Boil two pints of spring water, add it to the mixture, sweetened to taste, and add a large teacup of rum. Bottle the medicine and drink a teacupful every few hours. This "hardly ever fails."

Fingers, numbness

Take a handful each of red sage, red fennel and red nettle, mix them with bay leaves and long pepper (a flowering vine), and crush them all together in a mortar. Strain these herbs through a cloth with aqua vitae (a spirit such as brandy or whisky). Apply this liquor to the hands at bedtime.

Foot, pain

If a foot has been bruised or crushed, eat the root of a mugwort plant with honey "and it will ease the pain thereof."

Foot, swollen

Bathe your feet in water that elder leaves have been sodden in.

Headache (1)

Mix two spoonfuls each of rosewater, juice of chamomile, woman's milk and strong wine vinegar. Heat the liquid in a dish and soak a piece of dry rose cake in it. When it is hot and has absorbed the liquid, add to the cake two good spoonfuls of powdered nutmeg. Then break it in half and place the two pieces one on each side of the head and lie down to rest.

Headache (2)

Take vervain, betony, wormwood, tetterwort, rue, some bark of the elder tree, honey and pepper. Pound them all together and gently boil the mixture in water. Drink it early in the morning and late at night.

Headache (3)

Take the juice of rue (sometimes known as garden rue, or herb of grace), and place it in the nostrils. This is to remove phlegm and clear the brain. Rue sodden in wine does the same.

Headache (4)

Pound some rose cake in a mortar with a little ale. Dry it by heating it up and place it on the nape of the neck at bedtime.

Hearing, partial loss of

Make a round loaf full of sage. Bake it, and then cut it in half and, while it is as hot as you can stand, bind it to the ears. Do this three or four times, "and it will cause the patient so grieved to hear well."

Heart disease, relief of

Take equal quantities of sage and mint, and boil them gently in white wine. Make a plaster with the herbs and lay it next to the heart until the patient feels well. To improve the appetite of the patient, he or she may also drink a little of the wine that the herbs were boiled in, evening and morning.

Heart infection

Mix together a handful each of borage, langdebeef (bristly oxtongue – a type of daisy), and calamint, and half a handful each of hart's-tongue (a fern), red mint, violets, and marigolds. Boil them in white wine or water. Then add a little saffron and sugar, boil them again, and strain the liquor into a container. Take seven spoonfuls each morning and evening.

Heart sickness

Take a handful each of rosemary and sage, and gently boil the herbs in white wine or strong ale. The patient should drink this lukewarm.

Insomnia (1)

Mix together one dram of dried, powdered saffron, one dram of dried, powdered lettuce seeds, and two drams of dried, powdered white poppy seeds. Add a little woman's milk until it is as thick as a balm, and then stick it to the temples of the head. This will effect sleep, but have the balm removed after no more than four hours.

Insomnia (2)

Take some berries off a laurel tree, crush them in a mortar, and place them all around your head.

Insomnia (3)

Mix together a spoonful each of rosewater and vinegar, two spoonfuls of oil of roses, half a handful of dried rose leaves crushed into powder, and enough bread crumbs to make a balm. Place this on the forehead and temples.

Insomnia (4)

Warm the leaves of elder, and bind them to the nape of the neck. This "will make him to sleep."

Jaundice (1)

Take a large apple and cut the top off, but keep both parts of the apple. Take out and discard the core, then fill the hole with butter, a large amount of turmeric, and some saffron. Replace the top of the apple, roast it until it is very tender, and eat it over three or four mornings – or more if need be.

Jaundice (2)

Take a large handful of celandine leaves (or celandine roots in the winter), and boil them in two pints of white wine until the liquor has reduced to one pint. Drink this warm in the morning and evening.

Joints, aching

Fry together marshmallows, milk, linseeds, powdered cumin, the whites of eggs, saffron, and white grease. Place the balm on the aching joints. "This hath been proved."

Knees, aches or swellings (1)

Boil a handful of thyme and a good piece of butter in two pints of Malmsey (Greek fortified wine) until it is reduced to one pint. Just before bedtime bathe your knees in this liquid, and moisten a cloth in it. Heat the cloth as hot as you can stand, and place it around your knees overnight. Do this six or seven times "and it will doubtless help you."

Knees, aches or swellings (2)

Take two handfuls of lavender leaves, or the flowers, or both together. Crush them finely in a mortar, and soak the herbs for two hours in a pint of wine. Strain it through a cloth and boil the liquid. Then with a sponge bathe the aching or swollen knee over six days.

Knees, sore, aching or swollen

Make a balm out of crushed rue, lovage and honey, and apply it to the sore knees. Do this three or four times to remove the swelling and relieve aching.

Lactation

See **Breastfeeding**.

Legs, aching

Crush some sage, rue, wormwood, sorrel leaves, horehound and red nettles in a mortar. Then mix the crushed herbs thoroughly with butter, and let it stand for ten days. Fry the mixture a few times, and strain it clean. This may be applied to all manner of aches in the legs.

Melancholy

Boil together the juice of lemons and pippins (apples) with sugar. Take two spoonfuls in the morning and evening.

Memory, loss of (1)

Place some mugwort in white wine, and then distill it. Drink it on an empty stomach to preserve the memory.

Memory, loss of (2)

Grind mustard seeds and mix the powder with vinegar. Rub it hard on the soles of the feet to quicken the memory of those who have been ill. It is said that this will not only help to reduce their forgetfulness, but it will also improve their concentration.

Memory, loss of (3)

Mix together rue, mint, olive oil and vinegar, and inhale the fumes of this liquor.

Menstruation, excessive

Blanch half a pound of almonds and crush them in a mortar. Then add the yolks of 12 hardboiled eggs and pound them with the almonds. Stir in one pint of good, strong vinegar and put all of this into a sealed earthenware container. Take five or six spoonfuls of this medicine, warmed up, three or four times a day as required.

Mental faculties, impaired (1)

Put betony powder in your soup, stew or casserole to restore brainpower. The patient may also chew mace, or place a root of galangal in his or her nostrils to strengthen the brain and improve memory.

Mental faculties, impaired (2)

Extract by pounding in a mortar the juice of marigolds, sage and wormwood. Add one spoonful of each of the three liquids to three spoonfuls of white wine. Drink it cold in the evening and morning. Repeat for five days.

Mental faculties, impaired (3)

To quicken the wit and sharpen the memory, beat langdebeef (bristly oxtongue – a type of daisy) in a clean mortar. Drink the juice of this with some warm water to "find the benefit."

Migraine

Thinly slice four or five nutmegs and place them in two small linen bags. Then soak the bags in pure red rose water and heat them up. Place the bags on the temples of your head.

Muscle, ache

Boil in two pints of ale a handful each of parsley and wormwood, adding some butter. Wash the part of the body that aches with this mixture, and stick the herbs, as hot as possible, to the aching area.

Muscle, aches, bruises and strains

Mix together four pints of neatsfoot oil (an oil that can be purchased), two pints of ox gall, a pint of aqua vitae (spirit such as brandy or whisky), a pint of rosewater, and a handful each of crushed bay leaves, rosemary leaves, lavender, and strawberry leaves and roots. Boil it all gently but thoroughly in a two-gallon pan, and then let it stand until it is almost cold. Strain it through a coarse linen cloth, discarding the sediment, and seal the liquor in a glass container. Rub it on the affected area as and when required.

Nails, to make them grow

Mix together some wheat flower and honey to make a balm. Coat the nails with this "and it will help them."

Nose, running (1)

To stop excessive discharge from the nose (for dry phlegmatic humors), mix together dried, powdered sage, powdered sea salt, and finely grated nutmeg. Place them in a linen bag, heat it up, and hold it on the nape of the neck.

Nose, running (2)

To stop excessive discharge from the nose (for dry phlegmatic humors), follow the instructions for curing a weak stomach (see **Stomach, weak** below).

Palsy

Drink every morning half a pint of distilled lavender water, and rub the head vigorously every morning and evening with a very clean, coarse cloth. By doing this the humors are dissolved and dispersed to the outward parts of the body. Furthermore, you should keep your feet and the nape of your neck warm and dry to prevent pain from recurring.

Piles (1)

Crush either the small leaves of wormwood or the roots of daisies very finely. Add some English honey, and put the mixture into a linen cloth. Apply the balm to the sore place and leave it there until the pain has gone.

Piles (2)

Cut the core out of a large onion, fill the hole full of sugar, and plug the hole. Wrap the onion up and roast it. While it is still hot, place the onion on the affected area.

Sadness

See **Melancholy**.

Scurvy

Extract the juice from goosegrass (cleavers) and take three spoonfuls in the morning before breakfast and two spoonfuls at bedtime until you are well.

Skin blemishes, pimples (1)

Make a paste by mixing some wheat flour with vinegar and honey, and lay it upon the blemishes to clean and clear the skin.

Skin blemishes, pimples (2)

Stir together some rosewater and water of wild tansy (a common herb known also as golden buttons). Use this to wash your face.

Skin blemishes, pimples (3)

Make and apply an ointment made from lupin flowers and lemon juice.

Skin disease (tetter), ringworm, or itch
Mix together some salad oil and salt, and warm it slightly, then apply it to the affected area of the skin.

Skin, itchy
Pound some dock roots in a mortar, then fry them with fresh butter. Apply this balm to the affected area of the skin five or six times.

Skin, sore
To cure a burning sore, gently boil elder leaves in milk until they are soft. Then strain off the liquid and boil them again until the balm is thick. Apply it to the sore as necessary.

Skin, wrinkles (1)
Take the flowers of rosemary and boil them in white wine. Wash the face with this. If you drink this liquid it will also sweeten the breath.

Skin, wrinkles (2)
Mix together some white wine, a little bryony (a flowering herbaceous shrub), and a large dried fig. Apply this to the face, rubbing it vigorously.

Sleepiness (1)
Gently boil in one pint of water a whole garlic, together with the husk, until the liquid has reduced to one third. Drink the liquid.

Sleepiness (2)
Eat parsley and fennel together.

Stomach, upset
Take equal quantities of endives and mint, and put them in white wine for twenty-four hours. Then strain it, discarding the herbs

and keeping the liquor, add a little cinnamon and pepper, and drink it. To comfort the stomach even more, and to aid "swift and good digestion," add a little powdered horsemint and calamint.

Stomach, weak

To strengthen a weak stomach make and drink Hippocras (similar to mulled wine or glühwein, but stronger): Put a pint of aqua vitae (spirit such as brandy or whisky) in a container. Then beat together into a coarse powder two ounces of cinnamon, one ounce of ginger, and a quarter of an ounce each of cloves and nutmeg, and add them to the aqua vitae. Bottle it and shake it a few times every day for nine days. Add a spoonful of this to a glass of warm wine, or to half a pint of warm ale, and drink it.

Stones, kidney or spleen (1)

Distill some parsley water and add it to white wine or good ale. Drink this to destroy the stone. This is "A medicine not only to break the stone, but also clearly to purge you thereof, if you doe use the same daily."

Stones (2)

Mix together one ounce of distilled lemon juice (or alternatively two ounces of undistilled lemon juice) and three ounces of concentrated radish juice to clear the stone from the body.

Stones (3)

Mix one grated nutmeg with the yolk of a new-laid egg.

Stones (4)

Mix four ounces of refined sugar with four ounces of fennel seeds and eight ounces of syrup of althea (marshmallow).

Stones (5)

Cut up into fine bits some ginger and small, ripe lemons. Distill them in a glass alembic, and take three or four spoonfuls while fasting. This will "break the stone and the patient shall void the gravel."

Sunburn

Mix together the juice of lemons with a little sea salt. Wash your face with it, and let it dry naturally. Do this three or four times.

Sweating excessively

Crush linseed and lettuce in a mortar, apply it to the stomach, and leave it there for four hours.

Throat, sore

Add three spoonfuls of honey to one pint of water and boil them together. Remove and discard the scum and add to the liquid one ounce of raisins. Leave it to stand for a while, and then strain it well through a cloth. Drink it morning and evening.

Toothache (1)

Mix together half a handful each of sage, rue, celery (preferably wild), feverfew (*Tanacetum parthenium*), wormwood and mint, and pound them well. Add four drams of vinegar, one dram of sea salt, and a little aqua vitae. Stir them well together, then put the mixture in a linen pouch and heat it up as hot as you can stand. Place it on the side of the face affected and lie on that side. As it cools, heat it up again and repeat as necessary.

Toothache (2)

Put some strong ale, mustard and "gumme elder" (secreted sap from an elder tree) in a shallow dish and heat it up, stirring it until it is thick. Place it on the side of the face where the pain is.

Urination, difficulty with (1)

Mix together a quarter of a handful each of parsley and fennel, and wash and finely shred them. Put the herbs into a cup of stale ale, and make a posset with it by adding curdled milk. Drink it as required.

Urination, difficulty with (2)

Put some mallows and a good quantity of Gromwell (*Lithospermum*) in a pot, and boil them for a good while in vinegar. Drink the liquid warm.

Medicine making, then, is not as difficult as one might imagine; but the main ingredient that goes into preparing most of them is *time*. For this reason a selection of lotions and potions should ideally be made in advance of illnesses occurring. Thus, we might want to follow the example of household mistresses of yesteryear by making some "base" medicines to which other ingredients are added as and when they are needed. These are waters and syrups made from a variety of fruits and herbs. Two popular base medicines that were usually items in stock, and which feature in many medical recipes, are rosewater and lemon syrup. These may also be used as tonics. Recipes show that while fruit syrups are typically made by boiling together equal quantities of sugar and sliced or diced fruit, and then straining away the sediment and keeping the liquid, waters are made by concentrating or distilling the juice of herbs, flowers or fruits. Thus, useful items might be an alembic, a pestle and mortar (or a liquidizer), clean containers with tightly sealing lids, and fine sieves or cloth.

Lemon peel is humorally warm, and lemon seeds are even hotter; but the flesh and juice of the fruit – like rosewater – is cool and dry. So why have two medicines with similar humoral characteristics, both of which appear to be inducers of black choler? Basically, while the lemon's coldness cools fevers, and its dryness counters phlegmatic conditions, the lemon's astringency and sharpness cuts through corrupt humors and fights infections. The sugar in the syrup not only acts as a preservative, but just as importantly it also provides the humoral warmth and moisture that can counter melancholically induced illnesses. Rosewater, physician Tobias Venner tells us in his book *Via Recta ad Vitam Longam*, "please a weak stomacke, comfort the heart, temper and purifie the blood, expel sadness, and are enemies to melancholy." All roses, he notes, are predominantly cold in the first degree, and, being dried, "they doe binde and drie, and likewise coole." The sweet and pleasant "smell of Roses is very comfortable to all the senses, spirits, and principall parts of the bodie, and so is the distilled water of them, which doth also gently temper and coole the inward parts."

In summing up the medicinal value of the rose, Venner says that it removes surplus moisture from the body that would otherwise attract disease. But what about the apparent contradiction that cool, dry roses can be "enemies to melancholy"? After all, it is seeing apparent contradictions, and not seeing black and yellow bile, that discredits humorism in the eyes of some skeptics. The keyword here, though, is "apparent." Rosewater in Venner's day typically was made with red wine, and rose syrup was, and still is, made with sugar. Red wine, like sugar, is humorally warm and moist. Thus, by getting the relative quantities right, lemon- and rose-based medicines can inhibit the overproduction of black bile which itself can result in melancholy.

One can make alternative base medicines to these, and add other active ingredients mentioned in this chapter as and when required; but the best course of action, as experts on the humoral body have known and stressed for ages, is to follow a diet appropriate to one's own humoral makeup. It is hoped that Chapters Three to Seven have provided the reader with the information to make a start on this, and the list of further reading that follows will enable everyone so inclined to become experts on medical self-help.

Bibliography

All pre-modern books listed in this bibliography are available to read on the websites Early English Books Online (EEBO) and Eighteenth Century Collections Online (ECCO). These websites may be accessed for free at many of the main libraries in towns and cities.

A. T., *A rich store-house or treasury for the diseased* (London: Thomas Purfoot, 1596).

Anon, *Here begynneth a newe boke of medecynes* (London: J. Rastell, 1526).

Austen, Ralph, *A treatise of fruit-trees* (Oxford: William Hall, 1665).

Baker, Robert B. and McCullouch, Laurence B. (eds), *The Cambridge World History of Medical Ethics* (Cambridge: Cambridge University Press, 2009).

Baker, Thomas, *Reflections upon learning* (London: A. Bosvile, 1700).

Baley, Walter, *A briefe treatise touching the preservation of the eie sight consisting partly in good order of diet, and partly in use of medicines* (Oxford: J. Barnes, 1602).

Ball, John, *The female physician: or, Every woman her own doctress* (London: L. Davis, 1770).

Ball, John, *The Modern Practice of Physic* (London: A. Millar, 1762).

Blagrave, Joseph, *Blagrave's supplement or enlargement to Mr. Nich. Culpeppers English physitian* (London: Obadiah Blagrave, 1674).

Boorde, Andrew, *A compendyous regyment* (London: Wyllyam Powell, 1547).

Boyle, Robert, *Of the reconcileableness of specifick medicines* (London: Sam. Smith, 1685).

Bradwell, Stephen, *Helps for suddain accidents* (London: Thomas

Purfoot, 1633).

Bright, Timothie, *A Treatise, Wherein is Declared the Sufficiencie of English Medicines* (London: H. L., 1615).

Bruele, Gualtherus, *Praxis medicinae* (London: John Norton, 1632).

Buchan, William, *Domestic Medicine* (Waterford: James Lyon and Co., 1797).

Bullein, William, *The Government of Health* (London: Valentine Sims, 1595).

Burton, Robert, *The anatomy of melancholy: what it is* (London: John Lichfield and James Short, 1621).

Butts, Henry, *Dyets Dry Dinner* (London: Thomas Creede, 1599).

Cartwright, Thomas, *An hospitall for the diseased* (London: Edward White, 1579).

Chesne, Joseph du, *The Sclopotarie of Josephus Quercetanus, phisition* (London: Roger Ward, 1590).

Cheyne, George, *An Essay of Health and Long Life* (London: George Strahan, 1724).

Cogan, Thomas, *The Haven of Health* (London: Anne Griffin, 1636).

Crab, Roger, *The English Hermite* (London: s. n., 1655).

Croft, Robert, *Paradise within us: or, The happie mind* (London: B. Alsop and T. Fawcet, 1640).

Cromwell, Oliver, *His Excellencies order, to the severall colonels of the army, concerning provision of quarter, diet, physick and attendance for the sick souldiers of their severall regiments* (London: s. n., 1650).

Culpeper, Nicholas, *The English physitian* (London: Peter Cole, 1652).

Elyot, Thomas, *The castel of helth* (London: Thomas Bertheleti, 1595).

Estienne, Charles, *Maison Rustique* (London: Edmund Bollifant, 1600).

Fioravanti, Leonardo, *A short discours of the excellent doctour*, translated by John Hester (London: Thomas East, 1580).

Freedman, Paul, *Out of the East: Spices and the Medieval Imagination* (New Haven: Yale University Press, 2008).

Gerard, John, *The Herball or Generall Historie of Plantes* (London: Adam Islip, Joice Norton and Richard Whitakers, 1633).

Goeurot, Jean, *The Regimen of Life* (London: William How, 1578).

Gordon, D., *Pharmaco-pinax, or A table and taxe of the pryces of all usuall medicaments, simple and composed* (Aberdeen: Edward Raban, 1625).

Gratarolo, Guglielmo, *A direction for the health of magistrates and studentes* (London: William How, 1574).

Guillemeau, Jacques, *Child-birth or, The happy deliverie of women* (London: A. Hatfield, 1612).

Guy's Hospital, *Elements of the practice of physic* (London: Guy's Hospital, 1798).

Guybert, Philbert, *The charitable physitian*, translated by I. W. (London: Thomas Harper, 1639).

Hart, James, *Klinike, or The diet of the diseased* (London: John Beale, 1633).

Hester, John, *The pearle of practise* (London: Richard Field, 1593).

Hieronymus Brunschwig, *The noble experyence of the vertuous handy warke of surgeri* (London: Petrus Treueris, 1525).

Hippocrates, *Aphorismes*, Book 1, ed. J. van Heurne (London: 1655).

Hunter, Lynette, "Women and Domestic Medicine: Lady Experimenters, 1570–1620," in L. Hunter and S. Hutton (eds), *Women, Science and Medicine 1500–1700* (Stroud: Sutton, 1997).

Kent, Countess of, Grey, Elizabeth, *A Choice Manual, or Rare Secrets in Physick and Chirurgery* (London: W. I., 1653).

Langton, Christopher, *A very brefe treatise, ordrely declaring the principal partes of phisick* (London: Edward Whitchurche, 1547).

Laudan, Rachel, "Birth of the Modern Diet," *Scientific American* 283:2 (2000), pp. 76–81.

Leong, Elaine, "Making Medicines in the Early Modern

Household," *Bulletin of the History of Medicine* 82:1 (2008), pp. 145–68.

Leong, Elaine and Pennell, Sarah, "Recipe Collections and the Currency of Medical Knowledge in the Early Modern 'Medical Marketplace,'" in M. S. P. Jenner and P. Wallace (eds), *Medicine and the Market in England and Its Colonies, c.1450–c.1850* (Basingstoke: Palgrave, 2007), pp. 133–52.

Levens, Peter, *A right profitable booke for all diseases* (London: J. Roberts, 1596).

Lloyd, Paul, "Dietary Advice and Fruit-eating in Late Tudor and Early Stuart England," *Journal of the History of Medicine and Allied Sciences* 67:4 (2012), pp. 553–86.

Lloyd, Paul, *Food and Identity in England, 1540–1640* (London: Bloomsbury, 2015).

Lloyd, Paul, "Making Waterfowl Safe to Eat: Medical Opinion, Cookbooks and Food Purchases in Early Seventeenth-century England," *Food and History* 11:1 (2013), pp. 35–55.

Lowe, Peter, *An easie, certaine, and perfect method, to cure and prevent the Spanish sickness* (London: James Roberts, 1596).

Markham, Gervase, *The English house-wife* (London: Nicholas Okes, 1631).

Mediolano, Johannes de, *Regimen sanitatis Salerni*, translated by T. Paynel (London: B. Alsop and T. Fawset, 1634).

Moffett, Thomas, *Healths improvement* (London: Thomas Newcomb, 1655).

Moore, Philip, *The Hope of Health* (London: Iohn Kyngston, 1564).

Norden, John, *Vicissitudo rerum* (London: Simon Stafford, 1600).

Paracelsus, Philippus, *Paracelsus of the chymical transmutation, genealogy and generation of metals & minerals* (London: Richard Moon, 1655).

Parkinson, John, *Paradisi in Sole Paradisus Terrestris* (London: Humfrey Lownes and Robert Young, 1629).

Partridge, John, *The widowes treasure* (London: Edward Alde, 1588).

Pelling, Margaret, *The Common Lot: Sickness, Medical Occupations and the Urban Poor in Early Modern England* (London: Longman, 1998).

Pollock, Linda, *With Faith and Physic: The Life of a Tudor Gentlewoman, Lady Grace Mildmay, 1552–1620* (London: Collins and Brown, 1993).

Primerose, James, *Popular errours. Or the errours of the people in physic* (London: W. Wilson, 1651).

Rantzau, Henrik, *The English mans doctor*, translated by J. Harrington (London: Augustine Matewes, 1624).

Roach, Frederick A., *Cultivated Fruits of Britain* (Oxford: Blackwell, 1985).

Robinson, Lewis, *Every Man His Own Doctor* (London: J. Cooke, 1785).

Ruscelli, Girolamo, *The secretes... Containyng excellent remedies against divers diseases, woundes, and other accidents*, translated by Wyllyam Warde (London: John Kingstone, 1558).

Sadler, John, *The sicke womans private looking-glasse* (London: Anne Griffin, 1636).

Shackelford, Jole, *A Philosophical Path for Paracelsian Medicine* (Copenhagen: Museum Tusculanum Press, 2004).

Tissot, Samuel, *Advice with Respect to Health* (London: G. Paramore, 1795).

Turner, Robert, *Botanologica the Brittish Physician* (London: R. Wood, 1664).

Turner, William, *The first and seconde partes of the herbal* (London: Arnold Birckman, 1568).

Vaughan, William, *Approved Directions for Health* (London: T. Snodham, 1612).

Venner, Tobias, *Via Recta ad Vitam Longam* (London: Edward Griffin, 1620).

Walkington, Thomas, *The optick glasse of humors* (London: Iohn Windet, 1607).

Wood, Owen, *An alphabetical book of physicall secrets* (London:

John Norton, 1639).

Woolley, Hannah, *The accomplish'd lady's delight* (London: B. Harris, 1675).

Note to the Reader

Thank you for purchasing *Become Your Own Doctor: Lost Secrets of Humoral Healthcare Revealed*. My sincere hope is that you derived as much information and enjoyment from reading this book as I did researching and writing it. If you have a few moments, please feel free to add your review of this book at your favorite online site for feedback (Amazon, GoodReads, etc.). You may also visit my website: http://paullloyd.weebly.com

Paul Lloyd

AYNI
BOOKS

"Ayni" is a Quechua word meaning "reciprocity" – sharing, giving and receiving – whatever you give out comes back to you. To be in Ayni is to be in balance, harmony and right relationship with oneself and nature, of which we are all an intrinsic part. Complementary and Alternative approaches to health and well-being essentially follow a holistic model, within which one is given support and encouragement to move towards a state of balance, true health and wholeness, ultimately leading to the awareness of one's unique place in the Universal jigsaw of life – Ayni, in fact.

Find more books at
www.ayni-books.com

The Jacket Technique
Being free from your excess baggage, you can take the first step towards effortless living
Hans de Waard
Find a life that truly fits.
Paperback: 2012 978-1-78099-447-5 $19.95 £11.99
eBook: 2012 978-1-78099-448-2 $9.99 £6.99

Japanese Art of Reiki
Bronwen and Frans Stiene
The first practical Reiki book from the traditional Japanese perspective.
Paperback: 2005 978-1-90504-702-4 $19.95 £12.99
eBook: 978-1-84694-640-0 $9.99 £6.99

New Reiki Software for Divine Living
An Energetic Embodiment of Divine Grace
Brett Bevell
Reiki healing simplified into one powerful easy-to-use technique.
Paperback: 2013 978-1-78279-004-4 $16.95 £9.99
eBook: 2013 978-1-78279-003-7 $9.99 £6.99

The Reiki Sourcebook (revised ed.)
Bronwen and Frans Stiene
Popular, comprehensive and updated manual for novice, teacher and the general reader.
Paperback: 2009 978-1-84694-181-8 $24.95 £12.99
eBook: 978-1-84694-648-6 $9.99 £6.99

You Can Beat Lung Cancer
Using Alternative/Integrative Interventions
Carl O. Helvie, R.N., Dr.P.H.
Significantly increase your chances of long-term lung cancer survival by using holistic Alternative/Integrative interventions by physicians/ health practitioners.
Paperback: 2012 978-1-78099-283-9 $26.95 £15.99
eBook: 2012 978-1-78099-284-6 $9.99 £6.99